Animal Feed Science and Nutrition - Production, Health and Environment

Edited by Amlan Kumar Patra

Published in London, United Kingdom

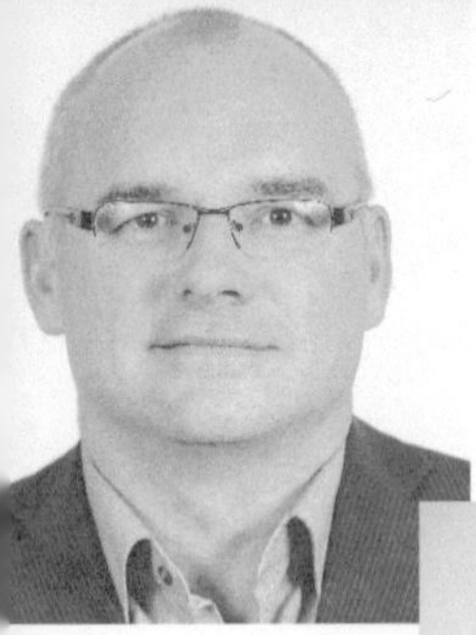
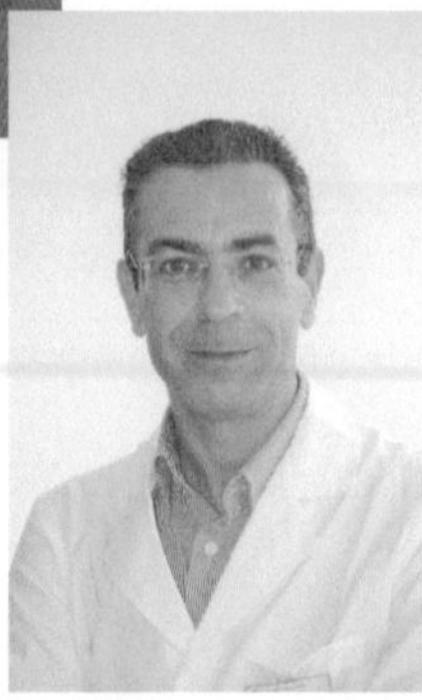
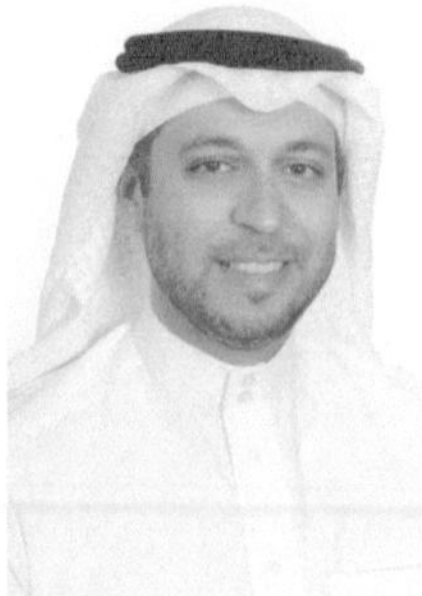
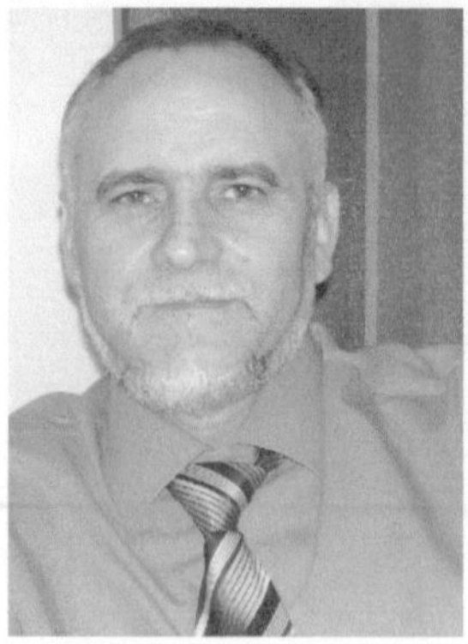
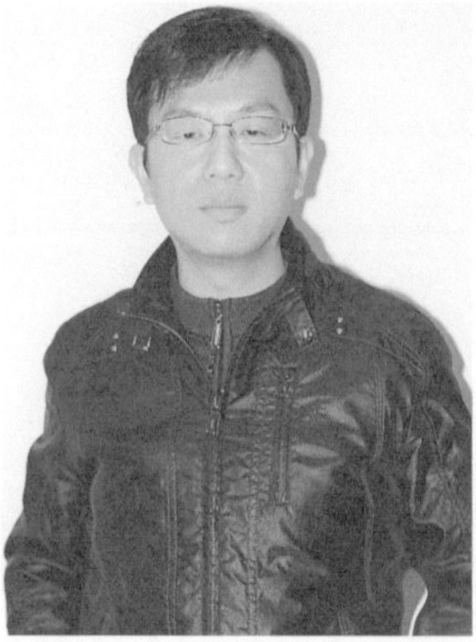
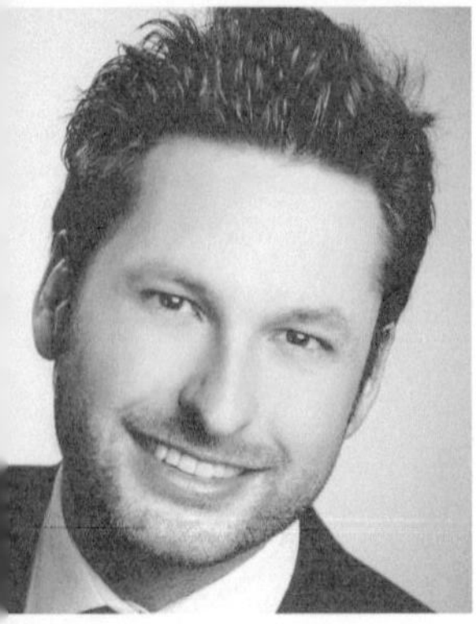
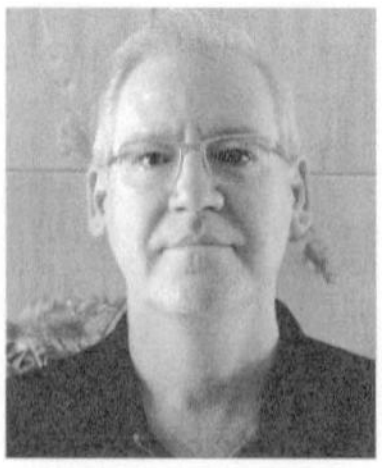

IntechOpen

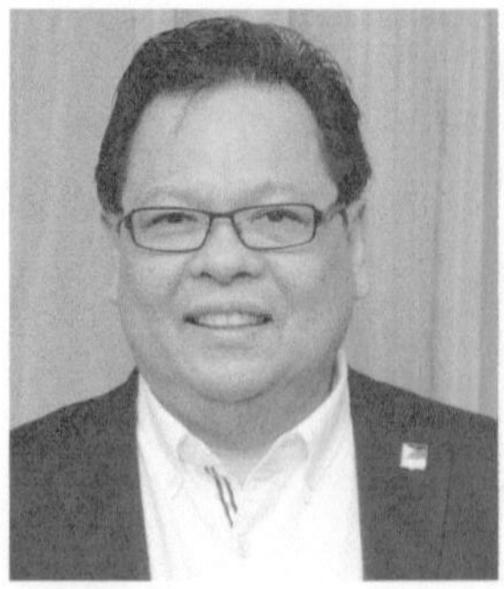
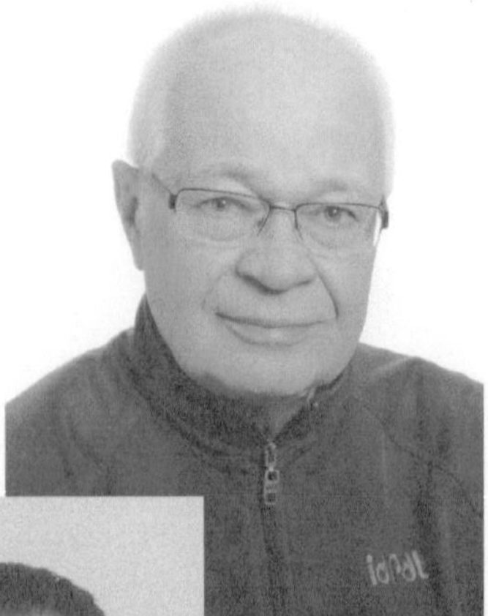
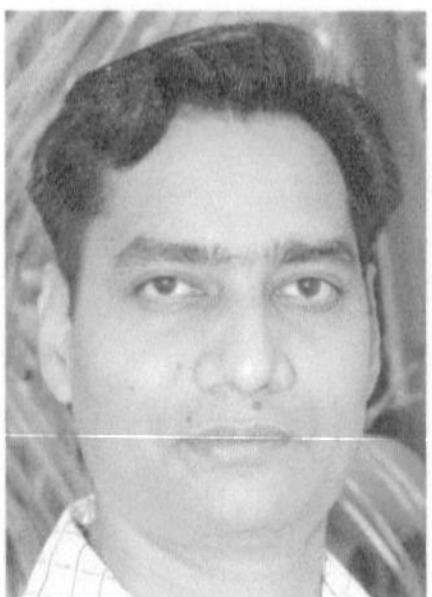
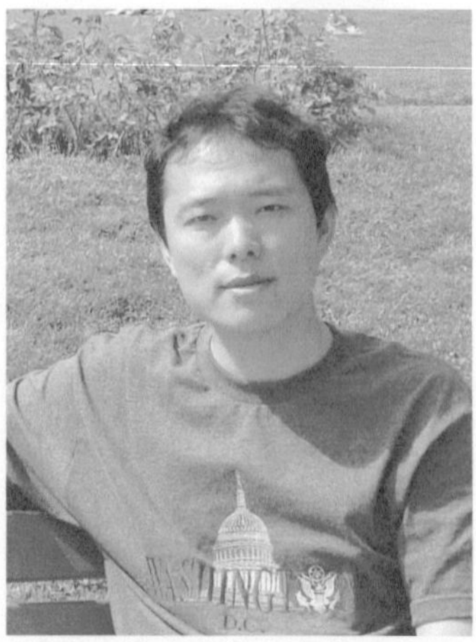
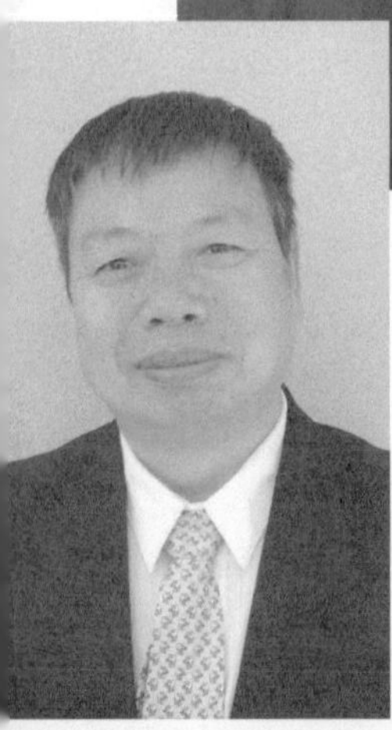
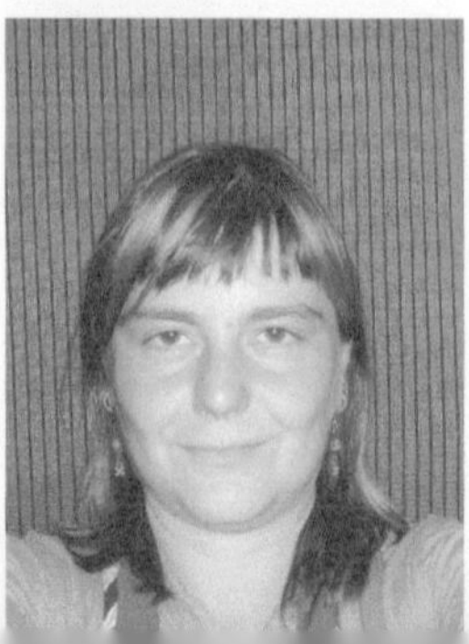

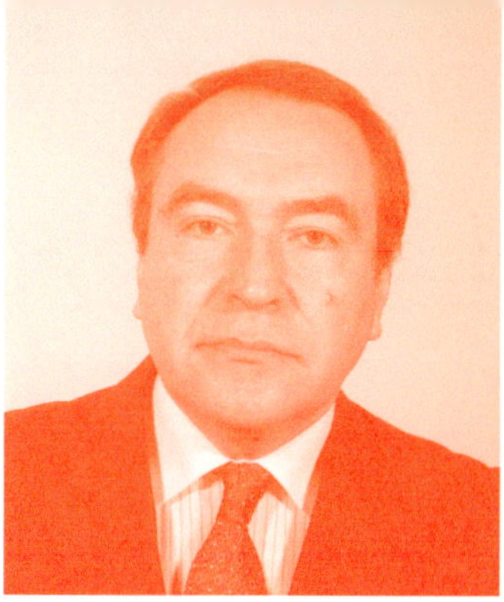
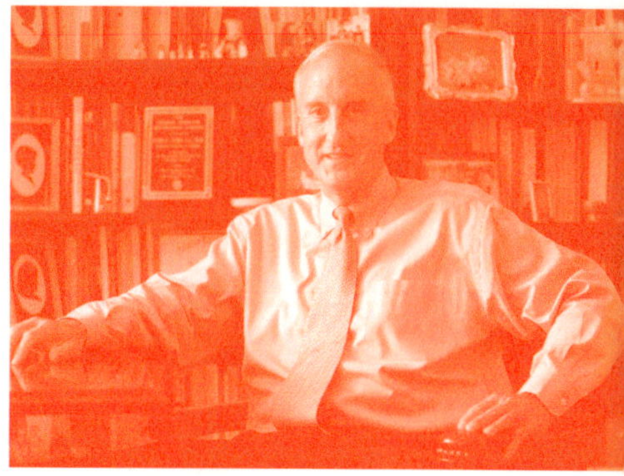
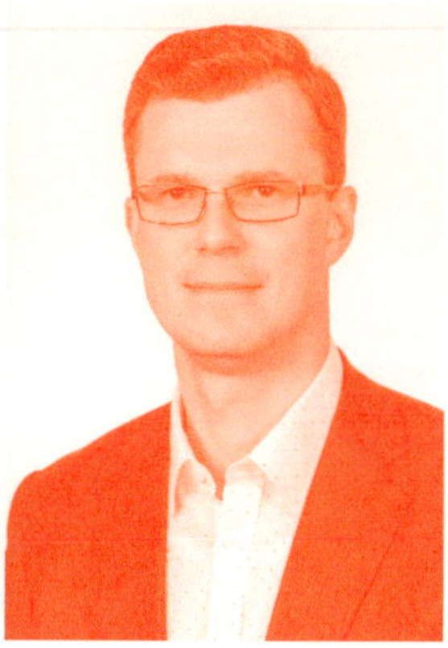
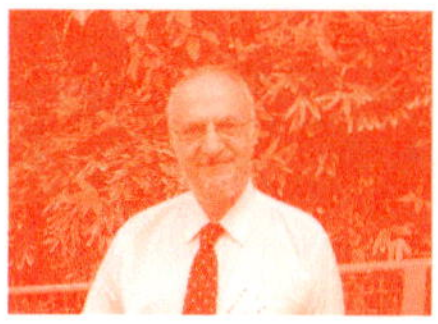
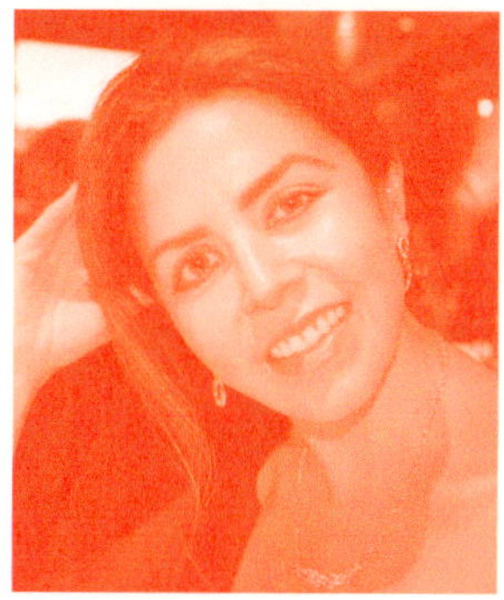

Supporting open minds since 2005

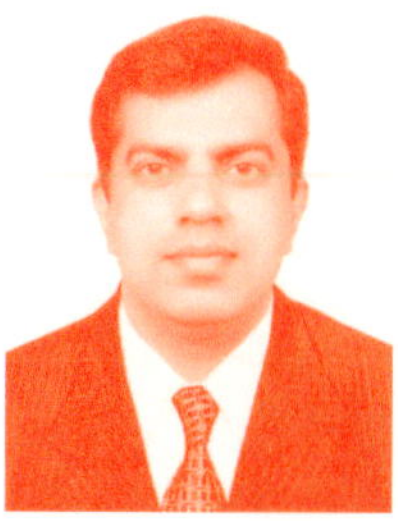
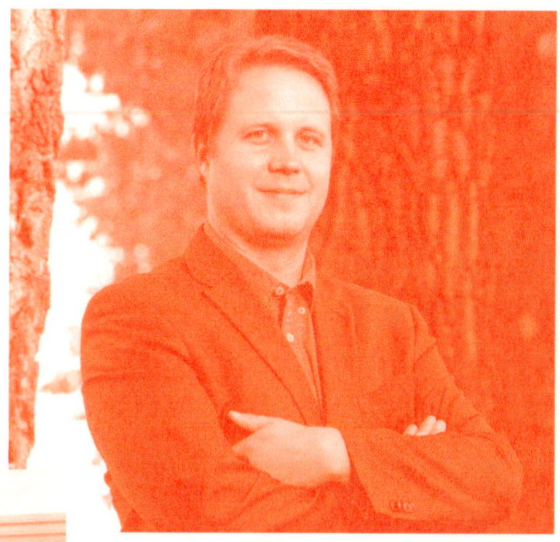
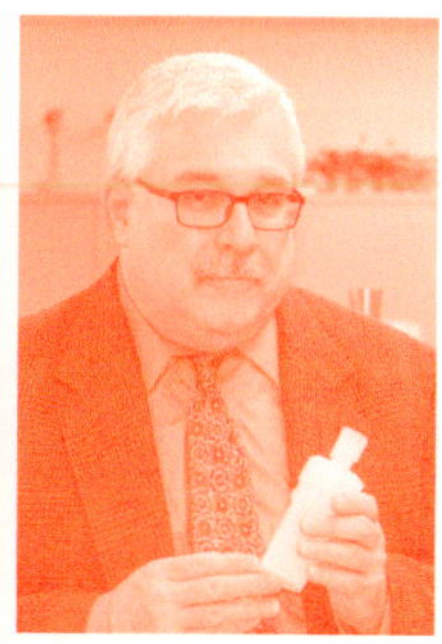
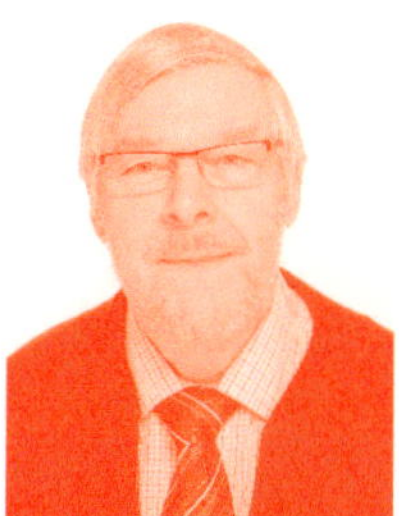
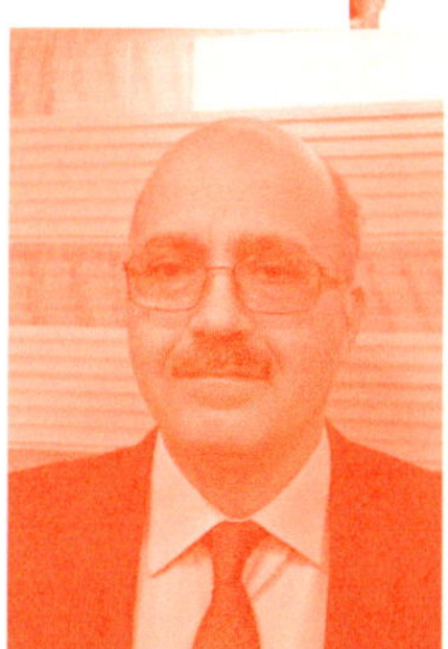
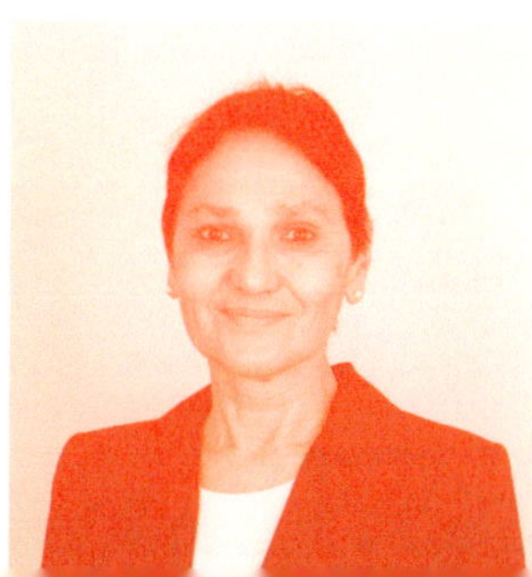
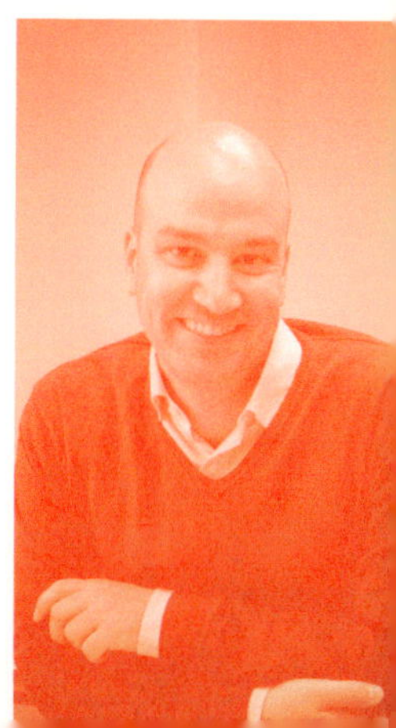

Animal Feed Science and Nutrition - Production, Health and Environment
http://dx.doi.org/10.5772/intechopen.95135
Edited by Amlan Kumar Patra

Contributors
Séga Ndao, Lipismita Samal, Sipho Moyo, Busani Moyo, Mardiati Zain, Rusmana Wijaya Setia Wijaya Setia Ningrat, Heni Suryani, Novirman Jamarun, Elieder Romanzini, Andressa Scholz Berça, Abmael Da Silva Cardoso, André Pastori D'Aurea, Lauriston Bertelli Fernandes, Ricardo Andrade Reis, Luís Eduardo Ferreira, Adesakin Taiwo Adekanmi, Amlan Kumar Patra, Yosra Soltan

First published in London, United Kingdom, 2022 by IntechOpen
IntechOpen is the global imprint of INTECHOPEN LIMITED, registered in England and Wales, registration number: 11086078, 5 Princes Gate Court, London, SW7 2QJ, United Kingdom
Printed in Croatia

British Library Cataloguing-in-Publication Data
A catalogue record for this book is available from the British Library

Additional hard and PDF copies can be obtained from orders@intechopen.com

Animal Feed Science and Nutrition - Production, Health and Environment
Edited by Amlan Kumar Patra
p. cm.

This title is part of the Veterinary Medicine and Science Book Series, Volume 10
Topic: Animal Nutrition
Series Editor: Rita Payan Carreira
Topic Editor: Manuel Gonzalez Ronquillo

Print ISBN 978-1-83969-860-6
Online ISBN 978-1-83969-861-3
eBook (PDF) ISBN 978-1-83969-862-0
ISSN 2632-0517

For EU product safety concerns:
IN TECH d.o.o., Prolaz Marije Krucifikse Kozulić 3, 51000 Rijeka, Croatia, info@intechopen.com or visit our website at intechopen.com.

IntechOpen Book Series
Veterinary Medicine and Science
Volume 10

Aims and Scope of the Series

Paralleling similar advances in the medical field, astounding advances occurred in the Veterinary Medicine and Science in recent decades, fostering a better support to animal health and more humane animal production, a better understanding of the physiology of endangered species, to improve the assisted reproductive technologies or the pathogenesis of certain diseases, where animals can be used as models for human diseases (like cancer, degenerative diseases or fertility), and even as a guarantee of public health. Bridging the Human, Animal and Environmental health, the holistic and integrative "One Health" concept intimately associates the developments within those fields, projecting its advancements into practice.
This book series aims to tackle a variety of fields in the animal-related medicine and sciences, providing thematic volumes, high quality and significance in the field, directed to researchers and postgraduates. It aims to give us a glimpse into the new accomplishments in the Veterinary Medicine and Science field. By addressing hot topics in veterinary sciences, we aim to gather authoritative texts within each issue of this series, providing in-depth overviews and analysis for graduates, academics and practitioners and foreseeing a deeper understanding of the subject. Forthcoming texts, written and edited by experienced researchers from both industry and academia, will also discuss scientific challenges faced today in Veterinary Medicine and Science. In brief, we hope that books in this series will provide accessible references for those interested or working in this field and encourage learning in a range of different topics.

Meet the Series Editor

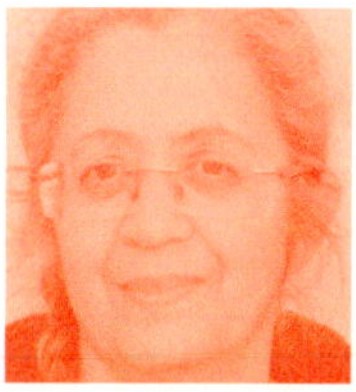

Rita Payan Carreira earned her Veterinary Degree from the Faculty of Veterinary Medicine in Lisbon, Portugal, in 1985. She obtained her Ph.D. in Veterinary Sciences from the University of Trás-os-Montes e Alto Douro, Portugal. After almost 32 years of teaching at the University of Trás-os-Montes and Alto Douro, she recently moved to the University of Évora, Department of Veterinary Medicine, where she teaches in the field of Animal Reproduction and Clinics. Her primary research areas include the molecular markers of the endometrial cycle and the embryo–maternal interaction, including oxidative stress and the reproductive physiology and disorders of sexual development, besides the molecular determinants of male and female fertility. She often supervises students preparing their master's or doctoral theses. She is also a frequent referee for various journals.

Meet the Volume Editor

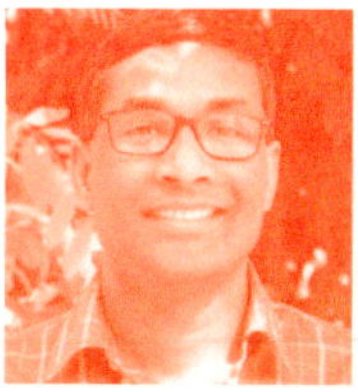

Amlan K. Patra, FRSB, obtained a Ph.D. in Animal Nutrition from Indian Veterinary Research Institute, India, in 2002. He is currently an associate professor at West Bengal University of Animal and Fishery Sciences. He has more than twenty years of research and teaching experience. He held previous positions at the American Institute for Goat Research, The Ohio State University, Columbus, USA, and Free University of Berlin, Germany. His research focuses on animal nutrition, particularly ruminants and poultry nutrition, gastrointestinal electrophysiology, meta-analysis and modeling in nutrition, and livestock–environment interaction. He has authored around 175 articles in journals, book chapters, and proceedings. Dr. Patra serves on the editorial boards of several reputed journals.

Contents

Preface XV

Section 1
Introduction 1

Chapter 1 3
Introductory Chapter: Animal Feed Science and Nutrition - Production, Health and Environment
by Amlan Kumar Patra

Section 2
Animal Production 11

Chapter 2 13
Advances in Pasture Management and Animal Nutrition to Optimize Beef Cattle Production in Grazing Systems
by Andressa Scholz Berça, Eliéder Prates Romanzini, Abmael da Silva Cardoso, Luís Eduardo Ferreira, André Pastori D'Aurea, Lauriston Bertelli Fernandes and Ricardo Andrade Reis

Chapter 3 37
Potential Utilization of Insect Meal as Livestock Feed
by Sipho Moyo and Busani Moyo

Chapter 4 55
Ruminal Microbiome Manipulation to Improve Fermentation Efficiency in Ruminants
by Yosra Ahmed Soltan and Amlan Kumar Patra

Section 3
Environment 75

Chapter 5 77
Analysis of Inputs Parameters Used to Estimate Enteric Methane Emission Factors Applying a Tier 2 Model: Case Study of Native Cattle in Senegal
by Séga Ndao

Chapter 6 95
Effect of Various Feed Additives on the Methane Emissions from Beef Cattle Based on an Ammoniated Palm Frond Feeds
by Mardiati Zain, Rusmana Wijaya Setia Ningrat, Heni Suryani and Novirman Jamarun

Chapter 7 113
Nutritional Interventions to Reduce Methane Emissions in Ruminants
by Lipismita Samal and Susanta Kumar Dash

Chapter 8 133
Health Hazards of Toxic and Essential Heavy Metals from the Poultry Waste on Human and Aquatic Organisms
by Adesakin Taiwo Adekanmi

Preface

The livestock production system faces several challenges including feed-food competition, shortage of high-quality feeds to support optimum potential performance, greenhouse gas emissions, environmental pollution, feed safety, feed-derived food safety, consumers' demands for better-quality animal-origin foods, and animal health and welfare. Some of these challenges may be further intensified in the future. As such, animal nutritionists and scientists are working to resolve potential threats to livestock production. This book begins with an introductory chapter highlighting these issues and their possible solutions, which may involve employing feeding and nutritional management in livestock production.

Optimum forage utilization in grasslands is necessary to fully exploit an animal's genetic potential. The book opens with an Introductory Chapter. Chapter 2 discusses tropical grassland management for grazing beef cattle for better utilization using supplementation of rumen undegradable protein and energy as well as dietary addition of alternative additives to antibiotics effects, such as probiotics, tannins, essential oils, and saponin, which can help to improve animal performance and nutrient utilization efficiency and decrease greenhouse gas emissions. Chapter 3 highlights the potential utilization of insect meal as a protein feed ingredient to economize rations and replace costly protein ingredients. It also discusses the benefits, safety, and acceptability of insect meals. Chapter 4 discusses how the improvement of ruminal fermentation efficiency could lead to better utilization of feeds (e.g., fiber-rich diets), lower greenhouse gas production, and improved quality of meat and milk.

An accurate approximation of methane emission factors and related variables is required for a better estimation of enteric methane emissions from livestock production systems. Chapter 5 analyzes the uncertainty and sensitivity of input parameters of enteric methane emission factors applying a tier 2 model with a case study of native cattle in Senegal. Chapters 6 and 7 describe different nutrition and feeding strategies including methane mitigation agents to lower methane production in ruminants. Chapter 8 delineates heavy metal pollution from poultry wastes and their health hazards in aquatic systems.

Overall, this book covers a wide area of challenges related to feed shortage, health, and environment in livestock production systems and their potential solutions. It is a useful resource for researchers and experts in animal production.

I would like to thank the authors for their excellent contributions. I would also like to thank Ms. Dolores Kuzelj at IntechOpen for her outstanding communications with the authors and myself throughout the editorial process of this book.

Amlan Kumar Patra
Department of Animal Nutrition,
West Bengal University of Animal and Fishery Sciences,
Kolkata, India

Section 1

Introduction

Chapter 1

Introductory Chapter: Animal Feed Science and Nutrition - Production, Health and Environment

Amlan Kumar Patra

1. Introduction

Different earth health indicators for "safe operating space," including degradation of land, climatic change, loss of biodiversity, deforestation, acidification of the ocean, and water scarcity, have deteriorated in recent decades, which is a great threat for the natural habitats along with human civilization [1]. Food animal production, which contributes significantly to gross domestic products in most of the countries of the world and provides nutritional and economic security of the farmers in low-income countries, has been recognized as significant divers of many ecological alterations in the Anthropocene period due to substantial share of greenhouse gas (GHG) emissions (methane and nitrous oxide) to the atmosphere [2]. Rapid increases in greenhouse gas (GHG) concentrations along with methane in the environment have become major drivers of climatic changes in the Anthropocene era [1]. Furthermore, food animal production faces many challenges, including shortage of high-quality feed ingredients, the contribution of pollutants to the environment, development of antimicrobial resistance due to inappropriate use of antibiotics and other antimicrobial chemical compounds, food safety, health, and welfare of animals. The demands of animal food products have risen sharply and will also increase considerably in the future owing to the growing human population, national economies, and urbanization. These changes will further intensify the challenges. The importance of animal feeding and nutrition is enormous in solving these challenges linked with food-fuel-feed competition, productivity, health and welfare, environment, product safety and quality [3]. In-depth analysis and better knowledge of the impacts of feeds and feeding on various domains of the livestock production systems focusing on the contribution of livestock in greenhouse gas emission, and providing solutions to challenges through improved technologies, policy, and institutional development measures are required [3]. In this chapter, some nutritional solutions to these challenges are described.

2. Identification of newer feed resources

Optimum potential performances of animals are not always expressed due to the improper supply of nutrients required for the physiological stages. This situation happens owing to the shortage of quality feeds for animals. Moreover, there is fuel-feed-food competition as feeds of livestock also include both human edible

IntechOpen

components and feedstock of biofuel production. With the increasing human population, human-edible feeds, such as cereal grains and soybeans, which constitute major ingredients for monogastric animals, may become less available for livestock. Maximum utilization of human-inedible feed ingredients will be required for sustainable livestock production. Many unconventional feeds have been identified to be used in the diets of different species of animals within specified limits. Some novel feed resources have been explored recently.

Several insect meals of different species are of interest recently as a protein source for monogastric animals due to their high protein composition and they are part of the natural diet of poultry. Insect meals could be sustainable protein feeds as they can be reared on low-grade biowastes, converting biowastes into high-quality protein sources. Amino acid composition and digestibility are promising, and studies have reported that insect meal can replace 50–100% soybean or fish meal depending upon animal species. The precise determination of amino acid digestibility and metabolizable energy content of different insect meals are required to properly balance the amino acids and energy in diets, particularly for monogastric species. It is technically possible to utilize insect meals as an alternative protein-rich feed ingredient [4].

Microalgae (green algae, blue-green algae, golden algae, and diatoms) are important marine resources and have the potential to become important sources of protein and bioactive compounds, vitamins, and minerals. Approximately, one-third of the world's total microalgae production is utilized for animal applications [4]. Microalgae can also be produced with waste materials, for example, manure and solar energy. The protein content of microalgae varies among species with a range of 25–50% [4]. Microalgae are also rich in n-3 long-chain polyunsaturated fatty acids, which would improve the meat and milk quality when they are used in diets of animals [5]. The cost-effective production of microalgae is a challenge.

Seaweed or macroalgae, for example, *Chlorophyta* (green algae), *Phaeophyceae* (brown algae), and *Rhodophyta* (red algae) contain up to 60% polysaccharides but are also rich in high-value compounds, such as n-3 fatty acids, bioactive compounds, and colorants. The nutritional composition of seaweeds shows a broad range, depending on the seaweed species. Brown macroalgae contain 5–13% crude protein and are rich in minerals, whereas red algae contain 10–30% of crude protein, and green algae over 15% crude protein [4]. Production of seaweeds faces some similar problems as microalgae. The composition of essential amino acids in most seaweed species is not optimal, and all seaweeds have high mineral content, which restricts their use in the diets of animals unless balanced properly [4]. Besides the potential use of seaweeds as feed ingredients, they have antimethanogenic effects in the rumen, which may be further beneficial environmentally [6].

The distiller's dried grains with soluble (DDGS) is a co-product from liquor and biofuel production. It contains high concentrations of protein and fats depending upon the grain stock used for ethanol production and can represent a valuable feed for livestock production. However, unlike cereal grains from which DDGS is derived, it mainly contains high amounts of low digestible fiber, such as cellulose, lignin, and arabinoxylans. Nonetheless, it may replace a certain amount of conventional costly feed ingredients and thus reduce the feed cost. Moreover, it contains fermented products with beneficial probiotic bacteria, prebiotics, enzymes, and bioactive metabolites to animals and thus could beneficially improve production performance [7].

Tree foliages are very useful fodder resources for small ruminant animal production, especially in the arid and semi-arid regions of the world, which provide supplementary proteins and micronutrients in low-quality forage-based diets [8]. Tree leaves may also be exploited to decrease greenhouse gas production and improve ruminal fermentation [9]. Residues from human-edible crops, vegetables and fruits, and food wastes can be utilized in all types of livestock diets that are usually fed to animals in low-income countries to some extent. The proper valorization of food wastes and residues of fruit and other processing industries as animal feeds is crucial for the transformation of the linear economy to a circular and sustainable bioeconomy, which will also reduce environmental burdens. The use of agro-industrial by-products in animal nutrition is a promising strategy to reduce the food-feed competition, the diet cost at the farm level, and the environmental impact of animal-derived food production. Moreover, many fruit and industrial wastes contain several medicinal and phytochemicals, which could be used to improve livestock production and health. The recent focus has centered on the use of plant secondary metabolites to improve ruminal fermentation, ruminant production, and health while minimizing the environmental burdens [10, 11].

3. Livestock and environment

Worldwide food production systems (livestock and vegetable-origin foods) contribute 18 Gt greenhouse gas (GHG; CO_2, methane, nitrous oxide, and fluorinated gases) emissions in CO_2 equivalent (CO_2e) (non-CO_2 gases are expressed as CO_2e based on the warming potential of the gases) account one-third (34%) of total global GHG based on detailed life cycle assessment analysis [12]. Different livestock activities, such as livestock rearing, feed production, land use and land-use change, manure management, transport, slaughtering, processing, and storage, contribute significantly to the total anthropogenic GHG emissions and are considered an important driver of global climate change in the food-system emissions. In livestock production, direct methane emissions from enteric fermentation and manure, and nitrous oxide emission during the process of nitrification and denitrification of the manure nitrogen comprise about 9% of total GHG emissions, and livestock share about 70% of total emissions from the agriculture, forestry and other land use [13]. Total direct non-CO_2 GHG emissions of enteric and manure sources globally increased from 1.77 Gt CO_2e in 1961 to 2.77 Gt CO_2e in 2010 at an annual growth rate of 0.92% [14]. Reduction of enteric methane emissions is needed to lessen the accountability of livestock production for GHG emissions. Different chemical inhibitors (e.g., halogenated methane analogs), defaunating agents and approaches, and ionophores (e.g., monensin) lower methanogenesis directly or indirectly in the rumen, but they do not exert consistent effects for practical uses. A range of nutritional strategies, such as increasing the cereal grains, feeding of leguminous forages containing high content of tannins, supplementation of low-quality roughages with readily fermentable carbohydrates and protein, and addition of fats with high concentrations of medium-chain fatty acids or long-chain unsaturated fatty acids, show promise for ruminal methane mitigation. Several new potential technologies, such as the use of plant secondary metabolites (polyphenols, essential oils, saponins, and alkaloids), propionate enhancers, bacteriocins, bacteriophages, probiotics, stimulation of acetogens, immunization, methane oxidation by methylotrophs, and genetic selection of low methane-producing animals, and development of recombinant vaccines targeting archaeal-specific genes, and cell surface proteins, have emerged to lower methane production [15]. Many plant secondary compounds, predominantly polyphenols, essential oils, saponins, and alkaloids, have been explored to modulate ruminal microbial fermentation and decrease methane production because of their antimicrobial and antimethanogenic properties [15]. Mitigation strategies of ruminal methane emission are considered to be less expensive than the reduction of CO_2 emission. Mitigation of methane emission by some technologies usually does not exert many negative results on ruminal fermentation but sometimes is associated with improved efficiency of animal production, which is beneficial in both environmental and nutritional perspectives. Many new technologies for methane mitigation have been explored, but only a few of them are practical and cost-effective, which can be adopted to accomplish mitigation of methane emissions at farm levels. A recent methane inhibitor, 3-nitroxypropanol, can significantly (up to 36%) lower enteric methane with some positive effect on milk component yield and body weight gain in cattle [16]. Different methane mitigation strategies in combination should be adopted to substantially mitigate methane emission from ruminants. The methane mitigation options that show both nutritional and environmental advantages would likely be better adopted by the farmers. For example, dietary fat up to 6% level could lessen methane emission moderately as well as improve animal productivity [17]. Similarly, nitrate supplementation could reduce the expensive protein meals in diets while decreasing methanogenesis. If some mitigation technologies could be employed to improve the nutritional values of forages, they would have immense practical importance in tropical feeding situations. However, mitigation of methane production is not consistent due to the adaptation of ruminal microbiota to the agents, dose, dietary composition, species, and production stages [18, 19].

Livestock species excrete an enormous amount of nitrogen and phosphorus to the environment with 92 Tg/year of nitrogen and 17 Tg/year of phosphorus in 2000, and this excretion is greater than nitrogen and phosphorus fertilizer use in croplands and grasslands [20]. Manure nitrogen excretion imparts a substantial share to the global nitrogen cycle, which is accountable for air pollution, water quality deterioration, climate change, and imbalances in biodiversity. The livestock production system shares approximately 40% of the total anthropogenic nitrous oxide and ammonia emissions globally, which arise from livestock manure nitrogen [21]. Dietary amendments are required by improving their utilization efficiency to reduce nitrogen and phosphorus excretion to the environment.

4. Feed safety, health, and welfare

Livestock feed represents the initial point of food safety in the farm-to-table supply chains. Therefore, the use of safe feeds is fundamental to human food safety. Feeds can contain inherent toxicants or can be contaminated with biological, chemical, and physical hazards during harvesting of the raw ingredients, manufacturing, processing, storage, or transport. In particular, pesticides, fungal toxins, and heavy metals are widespread in feedstuff. Heavy metal (e.g., cadmium, arsenic, lead, mercury, copper, and chromium) contents in feeds and water are particularly widely prevalent in industrial, urban, and semi-urban regions. Ultimately, animal-derived foods may contain high concentrations of these heavy metals, which is of public health concern. Therefore, contamination of the heavy metals in these regions needs special attention and preventive measures to reduce the heavy metal contents in meat and milk by nutritional amendments [22].

In-feed antibiotics are commonly added in the animal industry, but they are concerned about the development of antimicrobial-resistant pathogens, posing a possible danger to human health. Though different opinions have been stated on antibiotic resistance gene transfer from animal pathogens to human pathogens, a possible connection between the use of antibiotics at subtherapeutic levels and the antimicrobial resistance development among the microbiota has been reported in many studies [23]. Several alternatives have been explored in recent decades, which include probiotics, probiotics, synbiotics, organic acids, phytogenics, enzymes, antimicrobial peptides, bacteriophages, clay, and metals. These feed additives have better effects with respect to immunomodulation, gut health, and antioxidant status compared with antibiotics. Although the positive results of many of the alternatives have been well reported, there is a lack of clear knowledge on their mode of action, efficacy, and advantages and disadvantages of their applications [23].

Animals face different kinds of stresses, namely, overproduction, overcrowding, transportation, and temperature, which are welfare issues for the livestock production systems. The stresses reduce animal performance, immunity, deteriorate product quality, gut health, and increase vulnerability to diseases. Different stresses can be alleviated by proper feeding practices, such as the use of medicinal plants, gut microbiota-acting agents, and antioxidant vitamins and minerals, which can improve antioxidant status, gut health, and immunity in animals along with animal production and product storage quality [24]. Overgrowth of broiler chickens and turkeys predisposes to many metabolic diseases related to mainly cardiovascular (e.g., ascites and pulmonary hypertension syndrome) and musculoskeletal (e.g., lameness, dyschondroplasia, and spondylolisthesis) disorders resulting from high nutrient intake or high metabolic rate, which causes more economic loss than the infectious diseases [25]. In high-producing cows, subacute ruminal acidosis commonly occurs due to the feeding of high proportions of grains to balance the energy requirements, which reduces milk production, ruminal health, and barrier function [26].

5. Food quality

Consumers are increasingly interested in healthy foods, giving rise to increasing demand for foods with beneficial health and well-being effects. The concentration of many health-promoting fatty acids in milk and meat can be effectively enhanced through strategic feeding. Several studies have been targeted to decrease the concentration of saturated fatty acids, and to enrich the n-3 fatty acid and rumenic acid (cis-9, trans-11 C18:2) content in milk and meat. A wide variety of plant secondary compounds, including polyphenols (simple phenolic compounds, tannins, and flavonoids), essential oils, and saponins, which have specific antimicrobial effects in the rumen responsible for fatty acid biohydrogenation, has been investigated with varying success [27]. The effectiveness of essential oils and tannins is still inconsistent with some studies showing no beneficial effects and others a positive result on inhibiting the first step or, less commonly, the final step of biohydrogenation of polyunsaturated fatty acids [28, 29]. Plant secondary compounds with higher antioxidative properties may reduce volatile compounds, such as skatole and indole (responsible for off-flavor in meat), enhance antioxidant status, and decrease lipid peroxidation and deterioration of meat and milk quality during storage. Further research would be needed to unravel the causes of contradictory effects, which may be attributed to the diverse active compounds, ruminant animal species, dose, diet composition, and physiological stages [29].

6. Conclusions

The livestock production system faces several challenges, including feed-fuel-food competition, shortage of high-quality feeds to support optimum potential performance, greenhouse gas emissions, environmental pollution, feed safety, consumers' demands of better-quality animal-origin safe foods, antibiotic-resistant human pathogenic microorganisms, health and welfare of animals in recent decades. Some of these challenges may be further intensified in the future. Animal feeding and nutrition would play highly important roles in solving these challenges.

Newer feed resources, including valorization of biowastes, vegetable, fruit processing by-products as animal feeds, are required to replace human-edible feeds and to improve dietary quality by supporting optimum production. Proper feeding management can reduce greenhouse gas emissions and environmental pollution and enrich health-promoting bioactive principles in animal-derived foods while improving the health and welfare of animals.

Conflict of interest

The author declares no conflict of interest.

Author details

Amlan Kumar Patra
Department of Animal Nutrition, West Bengal University of Animal and Fishery Sciences, Kolkata, India

*Address all correspondence to: patra_amlan@yahoo.com

References

[1] Whitmee S, Haines A, Beyrer C, et al. Safeguarding human health in the Anthropocene epoch: Report of The Rockefeller Foundation–Lancet Commission on planetary health. The Lancet. 2015;**386**(10007):1973-2028

[2] Gerber PJ, Steinfeld H, Henderson B, et al. Tackling Climate Change through Livestock: A Global Assessment of Emissions and Mitigation Opportunities. Rome: Food and Agriculture Organization of the United Nations (FAO); 2013

[3] Makkar HP. Animal nutrition in a 360-degree view and a framework for future R&D work: Towards sustainable livestock production. Animal Production Science. 2016;**56**(10): 1561-1568

[4] Te Pas MF, Veldkamp T, de Haas Y, Bannink A, Ellen ED. Adaptation of livestock to new diets using feed components without competition with human edible protein sources—a review of the possibilities and recommendations. Animals. 2021;**11**(8):2293

[5] Madeira MS, Cardoso C, Lopes PA, et al. Microalgae as feed ingredients for livestock production and meat quality: A review. Livestock Science. 2017; **205**:111-121

[6] Min BR, Parker D, Brauer D, et al. The role of seaweed as a potential dietary supplementation for enteric methane mitigation in ruminants: Challenges and opportunities. Animal Nutrition. 2021;**7**(4):1371-1387

[7] Lalhriatpuii M, Patra AK. Feeding rice fermented beer waste improves growth performance, nutrient digestibility and nitrogen utilization in growing rabbits. Journal of Animal Physiology and Animal Nutrition. 2022;**106**:147-155

[8] Patra AK. Effects of supplementing low-quality roughages with tree foliages on digestibility, nitrogen utilization and rumen characteristics in sheep: A meta-analysis. Journal of Animal Physiology and Animal Nutrition. 2010;**94**(3):338-353

[9] Huang H, Szumacher-Strabel M, Patra AK, et al. Chemical and phytochemical composition, in vitro ruminal fermentation, methane production, and nutrient degradability of fresh and ensiled Paulownia hybrid leaves. Animal Feed Science and Technology. 2021;**279**:115038

[10] Singh P, Hundal JS, Patra AK, Wadhwa M, Sharma A. Sustainable utilization of *Aloe vera* waste in the diet of lactating cows for improvement of milk production performance and reduction of carbon footprint. Journal of Cleaner Production. 2021;**288**:125118

[11] Singla A, Hundal JS, Patra AK, Wadhwa M, Nagarajappa V, Malhotra P. Effect of dietary supplementation of *Emblica officinalis* fruit pomace on methane emission, ruminal fermentation, nutrient utilization, and milk production performance in buffaloes. Environmental Science and Pollution Research. 2021;**28**(14): 18120-18133

[12] Crippa M, Solazzo E, Guizzardi D, Monforti-Ferrario F, Tubiello FN, Leip A. Food systems are responsible for a third of global anthropogenic GHG emissions. Nature Food. 2021;**2**(3): 198-209

[13] Tubiello FN, Salvatore M, Rossi S, Ferrara A, Fitton N, Smith P. The FAOSTAT database of greenhouse gas emissions from agriculture. Environmental Research Letters. 2013;**8**(1):015009

[14] Patra AK. Trends and projected estimates of GHG emissions from Indian livestock in comparisons with GHG

emissions from world and developing countries. Asian-Australasian Journal of Animal Sciences. 2014;**27**(4):592

[15] Patra AK. Enteric methane mitigation technologies for ruminant livestock: A synthesis of current research and future directions. Environmental Monitoring and Assessment. 2012;**184**(4):1929-1952

[16] Melgar A, Welter KC, Nedelkov K, et al. Dose-response effect of 3-nitrooxypropanol on enteric methane emissions in dairy cows. Journal of Dairy Science. 2020;**103**(7):6145-6156

[17] Patra AK. The effect of dietary fats on methane emissions, and its other effects on digestibility, rumen fermentation and lactation performance in cattle: A meta-analysis. Livestock Science. 2013;**155**(2-3):244-254

[18] Patra AK, Yu Z. Effects of adaptation of in vitro rumen culture to garlic oil, nitrate, and saponin and their combinations on methanogenesis, fermentation, and abundances and diversity of microbial populations. Frontiers in Microbiology. 2015;**6**:1434

[19] Patra A, Park T, Kim M, Yu Z. Rumen methanogens and mitigation of methane emission by anti-methanogenic compounds and substances. Journal of Animal Science and Biotechnology. 2017;**8**(1):1-18

[20] Bouwman L, Goldewijk KK, Van Der Hoek KW, et al. Exploring global changes in nitrogen and phosphorus cycles in agriculture induced by livestock production over the 1900-2050 period. Proceedings of the National Academy of Sciences. 2013; **110**(52):20882-20887

[21] Oenema O, Wrage N, Velthof GL, van Groenigen JW, Dolfing J, Kuikman PJ. Trends in global nitrous oxide emissions from animal production systems. Nutrient Cycling in Agroecosystems. 2005;**72**(1):51-65

[22] Kar I, Patra AK. Tissue bioaccumulation and toxicopathological effects of cadmium and its dietary amelioration in poultry—a review. Biological Trace Element Research. 2021;**199**:3846-3868

[23] Lillehoj H, Liu Y, Calsamiglia S, et al. Phytochemicals as antibiotic alternatives to promote growth and enhance host health. Veterinary Research. 2018;**49**(1):1-18

[24] Patra AK, Kar I. Heat stress on microbiota composition, barrier integrity, and nutrient transport in gut, production performance, and its amelioration in farm animals. Journal of Animal Science and Technology. 2021;**63**(2):211

[25] Julian RJ. Production and growth related disorders and other metabolic diseases of poultry—a review. The Veterinary Journal. 2005;**169**(3):350-369

[26] Aschenbach JR, Zebeli Q, Patra AK, Greco G, Amasheh S, Penner GB. Symposium review: The importance of the ruminal epithelial barrier for a healthy and productive cow. Journal of Dairy Science. 2019;**102**(2):1866-1882

[27] Roy A, Mandal GP, Patra AK. Evaluating the performance, carcass traits and conjugated linoleic acid content in muscle and adipose tissues of Black Bengal goats fed soybean oil and sunflower oil. Animal Feed Science and Technology. 2013;**185**(1-2):43-52

[28] Patra AK. Exploring the benefits of feeding tannin containing diets for enhancing the nutritional values of milk and meat of ruminants. Indian Journal of Animal Health. 2014;**53**(2):63-76

[29] Toral PG, Monahan FJ, Hervás G, Frutos P, Moloney AP. Modulating ruminal lipid metabolism to improve the fatty acid composition of meat and milk. Challenges and opportunities. Animals. 2018;**12**(s2):s272-s281

Section 2

Animal Production

Chapter 2

Advances in Pasture Management and Animal Nutrition to Optimize Beef Cattle Production in Grazing Systems

Andressa Scholz Berça, Eliéder Prates Romanzini, Abmael da Silva Cardoso, Luís Eduardo Ferreira, André Pastori D'Aurea, Lauriston Bertelli Fernandes and Ricardo Andrade Reis

Abstract

The increasing demand of meat requires the adoption of sustainable intensification livestock systems, applying nutritional strategies to reduce any negative contribution from beef cattle to global warming and, at the same time, to increase animal performance and productive efficiency. The pasture management practices and feed supplementation, mainly using non-edible feed with less costs, could minimize environmental and social impacts, resulting in higher productivity with less inputs utilization. Tropical grass submitted to grazing management according to plant height present high soluble protein and low levels of indigestible neutral detergent fiber contents. Energy or rumen undegradable protein supplementation, associated to alternative additives to antibiotics effects, such as probiotics, tannin, essential oils and saponin, can help to fully exploit the animal genetic potential and nutrient utilization efficiency, which decreases greenhouse gases emissions and improves animal performance. Hence, more information about these tools can make the livestock systems in tropical pasture more efficient and eco-friendlier.

Keywords: greenhouse gases, non-edible feed, organic feed additive, supplementation, tropical pastures

1. Introduction

The large territorial extension and the tropical climate favorable to the growth of tropical grasses make pastures the basis for feeding Brazilian beef cattle, being the most practical and economical source to feed cattle in Brazil [1], responsible for the production of 89% of the entire herd, which reaches almost 188 million heads [2].

The economy globalization induces agriculture to become more and more efficient and competitive, therefore, failures in pasture management can be decisive in the success or unsuccess of beef cattle livestock [3]. In this sense, the great challenge of beef cattle production systems on pastures is the use of practices capable to increase the productivity and quality of meat with low environmental impact [4, 5]. For this, enhancing the animal performance and optimizing the use of basal forage resources is the main objective of management strategies to be adopted [6].

In Central Brazil, tropical forages present as a typical characteristic the seasonality of production, concentrating its growth between 70 and 80% in the rainy season, and 20 to 30% in the dry season [7]. The effects of this seasonality in beef cattle are evident through drastic variations in the chemical and structural composition of the forage canopy, which directly reflect on intake, digestibility, and weight gain and, consequently, delay the slaughter age of the animals [8]. The rainy season presents advantages for ruminant production as it has favorable edaphoclimatic conditions for the green leaf and forage mass productions with higher levels of crude protein (CP) and total digestible nutrients (TDN), when compared to the dry season, in addition to be the time to explore the maximum of animal performance and gain per area [9].

In theory, high-quality tropical forages should be able to provide the nutrients needed to meet grazing animals' requirement, including energy, protein, minerals and vitamins. However, the chemical composition of tropical grass forage is rarely in a state of balance between animal requirements and the nutrients needed to obtain high weight gains, due to the quantitative and qualitative seasonality inherent to the pasture system, interfering in the expression of the genetic potential of beef cattle in Brazil [10]. In this sense, the management strategies adopted by the manager can provide differences in the magnitude of responses in animal performance and weight gain per explored pasture area [11].

The intensification of the production system requires, in addition to the use of pasture management techniques, the adoption of nutritional strategies, such as the diet supplementation of grazing cattle, as well as the use of the genetic potential of the animals, through selection and crossings. Such strategies must be consolidated in order to ensure the profitability of the production system, sustainability of the pasture ecosystem and production of quality meat for the consumer market [5, 6]. Faced with such conditions, the search for alternatives to chemical additives that reduce the negative contribution of livestock to global warming and, at the same time, increase performance and productive efficiency is increasing [12]. In this context, the use of organic additives has been established, among these components are condensed tannins, saponins and essential oils. These compounds come from plants, usually its extracts, and have the ability to manipulate ruminal fermentation and animal metabolism, in order to increase performance and promote beneficial effects to the environment [13].

Therefore, this chapter aimed to address aspects related to the production of beef cattle from a sustainable perspective, considering grazing management, the strategic use of diet supplementation for grazing animals, featuring the inclusion of non-edible feed and organic additives on supplement composition and their results.

2. Aspects related to beef cattle in grazing systems

2.1 Livestock contribution to greenhouse gases

As the largest land use system in Brazil, the agricultural sector contributes 40% of the global agricultural gross domestic product, provides income for more than 1.3 billion people and food for at least 800 million people, using vast areas of pasture and a third of agricultural land for food production in the world [14]. However, although it assumes great importance in the economic scenario and is essential for world food, the rapid population growth and the production and consumption of agricultural products is contributing to a substantial emission of greenhouse gases (GHG) to the environment, being responsible for 14.5% of the total human induced GHG emissions in the world [15], which makes the activity often cited as the villain of global warming [16].

Livestock contributes to GHG emissions in the form of methane (CH_4) from enteric fermentation, nitrous oxide (N_2O) from the use of nitrogen (N) fertilizers, and CH_4 and N_2O from animal excreta management and deposition. Furthermore, carbon dioxide (CO_2) is also produced from the use of fossil fuel and energy on farms [5].

The production of enteric CH_4 by ruminants is a fundamental process for the adequate functioning of the digestive system of these animals, but it results in a loss of gross ingested energy and, consequently, reduces animal performance [16], in addition to having its contribution in 3.5% of the world's total GHG emissions [17]. Worldwide, CH_4 is considered the second largest contributor to global warming (16%), right after CO_2 (65%) [17]. The gas from livestock systems originates mainly from enteric fermentation (90%), being the rest produced from the fermentation of animal organic waste [18].

The use of N fertilizers and the deposition of animal excreta (feces and urine) are the main responsible for the losses of N to the environment, causing not only economic losses, but also environmental ones, due to nitrate leaching, volatilization of ammonia (NH_3) and, mainly, N_2O emission [19]. It is estimated that the annual global losses of N via excreta represent almost 26 million tons, and N fertilizers, 17 million tons [20]. The Intergovernmental Panel on Climate Change [17] estimates NH_3 volatilization values of 30% (20–50%) of excreta (urine and feces) and 15% (3–43%) of the urea fertilizer.

Although ruminants contribute with gas emissions to the environment, management strategies are essential for the sustainability of the global food system. In general, the practices involve improving the environmental performance of livestock systems through the management, supplementation, and adequate use of alternative additives to antibiotics; establish sustainable levels of intake of foods of animal origin, as well as using ingredients that are not consumed by humans (non-edible feed) [21, 22].

Indications for reducing CH_4 production include measures that reflect better animal performance and result in shorter production cycles, involving improvement in the composition and quality of forage, by reducing the cell wall and increasing levels of soluble protein and carbohydrates, e.g., improvement of animal genetics, feed supplementation [23]. Furthermore, the use of substances such as additives composed of organic acids, yeast and plant extracts, such as tannin and saponin, also help to reduce methanogenesis by manipulating ruminal fermentation [22].

A common strategy to reduce N losses in the system, both directly through N excretion via feces and urine, and indirectly through the use of fertilizers, is the mixed pastures of grass and legume, due to its association with nitrogen-fixing bacteria, which increases forage productivity and nutritive value [19]. The improvement in the diet quality, in turn, can change the urine and feces composition and, consequently, N losses through excreta [24].

2.2 Grazing management

Animal performance in pastures is mainly determined by forage quality, which is a function of dry matter (DM) intake and forage nutritive value [8]. In turn, the nutritive value is determined by the chemical composition and the nutrients directly responsible for the DM digestibility, CP and neutral detergent fiber (NDF) contents [8]. In this sense, the correct management of pastures affects both pasture chemical composition and structure, in addition to factors such as forage mass, supply of leaves, stem and dead material, which are determinants in the animal ingestive behavior and, consequently, in the nutrient's intake [25].

During the rainy season, the management must be done through strategies that guarantee the longest duration in the supply of quality forage and/or the improvement of forage nutritive value, aiming to achieve greater productivity of the system [26]. In this sense, pasture management should prioritize the adjustment in grazing intensity to obtain high yields per animal and per area, considering the morpho-physiological principles that govern the plant growth and its biological limits, in order to allow persistence of the pasture and avoid its degradation [12]. Any management criteria to be adopted, therefore, must consider the adjustment of forage allowance and stocking rate in order to simultaneously control the quality and quantity of available forage and maintain the sustainability of the system [11].

In general, pasture management involves a set of practices aimed at changing the morphology or delaying plant maturity, in order to increase the level of digestible nutrients in the diet for cattle and ensure adequate performance [27]. Furthermore, Sollenberger et al. [28] reported that grazing management should allow for a balance between plant growth, intake, and animal production, to keep a stable production system.

According to Pereira et al. [29], the control of pasture defoliation is crucial to the sustainability of the system, as it is an antagonistic event, that is, the plant uses the leaves to capture light and carry out photosynthesis, producing carbohydrates that allow the maintenance of life and of development. On the other hand, the leaf is the morphological component with the highest nutritive value that compose most of the diet of grazing animals [25]. Therefore, it is necessary to adopt management techniques that prioritize the forage plant and the grazing animal, allowing high forage productivity combined with high animal performance [5].

2.2.1 Grazing height

Pasture management based on the adjustment of grazing intensity can be done following several criteria, such as grazing pressure, forage allowance, residual forage mass, residual leaf area index (LAI), height, and others [11]. The adoption of height as a management criterion allows the control of forage mass and stocking rate, being able to relate pasture growth with its use and, consequently, with the canopy structure and responses in intake and animal performance [30]. In addition, height is a functional and practical field indicator, which can be correlated to other management criteria, such as forage allowance and light interception (LI) [31]. Also, grazing height directly affects the ingestive behavior of grazing animals [5].

According to Reis et al. [8], grazing management must adjust the frequency and intensity of defoliation, so that the animal can harvest forage at the appropriate physiological age, which directly affects the nature and concentration of structural carbohydrates in the cell wall and nitrogenous compounds, which are the main determinants of forage quality. Thus, the authors report that pastures kept under continuous stocking and efficiently managed can provide continuous intake of young leaves and, consequently, greater forage digestibility when compared to the intermittent stocking system.

Pasture management under different grazing intensities promotes different responses in forage mass accumulation and nutritive value. Studies conducted at FCAV/Unesp Campus de Jaboticabal, Brazil generated consistent data on the effects of different heights of tropical pasture management in the rainy season [30, 32–37]. The afore mentioned authors evaluated Marandu grass pastures in a continuous stocking and variable stock grazing system, at three heights: 15, 25 and 35 cm. As the grazing height increased, there was a reduction in CP and an increase in fiber contents, higher senescence rate and higher leaf elongation rate, the latter two being related to higher LAI, which intercepts a greater amount of solar radiation. On the other hand, canopies kept at a lower height showed reduced growth and senescence, lower forage accumulation, and restriction in the green material allowance, which limited intake and animal performance. In summary, the authors concluded that Marandu grass pastures managed under continuous stocking, during the rainy season, should be managed at 25 cm height, in order to maximize forage intake and individual daily weight gain in the growing phase, without a marked decline in weight gain per area.

In this sequence of studies, Marandu grass pastures managed under continuous stocking at 25 cm height corresponded to 95% of LI and, according to Delevatti et al. [38], this management results in pastures with a higher proportion of leaves, higher protein fraction, lower proportions of dead material and insoluble neutral detergent fiber (iNDF).

In Marandu grass pastures subjected to rotational grazing, 95% LI values during regrowth were also obtained with an average sward pre-grazing height of around 25 cm [39, 40]. According to Pedreira et al. [40], the management strategy of entering animals at 95% LI reduces the amount of self-shadowed material in the canopy and, therefore, reduces tissue death. Furthermore, in a rotational system, the height of the post-grazing residue interferes in the pasture intake due to changes in the canopy structure and the stratum explored by the animals during grazing [39].

2.2.2 Nitrogen fertilization

According to Reis et al. [11], the growth, development and chemical composition of forages are determining factors in animal performance, and, in turn, are affected by physiological aspects inherent to the plant and environmental conditions. Thus, N is the most limiting element for the development of forage grasses, due to the amount of nutrient extracted by the plant and the low residual effect of N in the soil after its application, also to losses through volatilization, leaching and immobilization by microorganisms [41].

In this scenario, the use of fertilization in pastures has been intensified in recent years, aiming to increasing the forage nutritive value and the stocking rate, which, consequently, increases the production per unit of area [38]. The pasture stocking rate, in turn, depends directly on the productivity of the forage plant, which is affected by several factors such as precipitation, temperature, light intensity, soil fertility and fertilization, especially with N [42].

According to Rezende et al. [43], the effect of N fertilization on yield is related to the initial tillering after cutting, as it promotes rapid expansion of the leaves, quickly replenishing photosynthetic tissues and increases tillers formation, responsible for higher DM production. In addition, N fertilization increases the concentration of CP, decreases N insoluble in neutral detergent and allows for greater efficiency in the rumen microbiota cellulolytic activity, factors that optimize animal performance [6]. The efficiency of N utilization by forage plants, however, is quite divergent, ranging from 5 to 89.2 kg of DM/kg of N applied [44].

The CP ruminal degradability of tropical and temperate forage plants is naturally high and increases with increasing N dose applied to the pasture [6]. Specially in tropical grass pasture management situations in which the high degradability of N compounds associated to the high content of structural carbohydrates with slow degradation is observed, the lack of balance between N and carbon skeletons arising from the degradation of carbohydrates in the rumen, compromises efficiency of nitrogen use (ENU) and microbial protein synthesis [45]. This condition, however, generates excessive losses of N compounds in the ruminal environment in NH_3 form in the urine, generating a protein deficit in relation to the requirements for high gains [9], which, in addition to resulting in economic losses, can be harmful to the environment through N losses in the form of volatilized NH_3, N_2O emission and nitrate leaching [4, 46].

In summary, pasture management practices during the rainy season, including maintenance N fertilization, adjustment in stocking according to the amount of forage available, provide pasture persistence, which surely dilutes production costs and gas emissions resulting from the inadequate land use and the prolonged period of pasture use [8].

2.3 Diet supplementation

In intensive production systems, supplementation is adopted as a technological tool to enhance the pastures use, aiming a compatible production with the genetic merit of the animals and profitability [27]. In general, supplementation allows the production of earlier animals, the increase in pastures support capacity, higher gain per animal and per area, the reduction of the time needed to reach slaughter weight, which, consequently, shortens the rearing and finishing grazing animals, in addition to the production of better-quality meat and carcass [9].

Thus, there is an increase in livestock offtake rates and a rapid turnover of invested capital, improving the efficiency and profitability of this system [47]. Furthermore, in grazing management systems that aims to optimize performance per animal and per area, it is possible to minimize the environmental impacts of beef cattle production in tropical grass pastures [4, 48].

The amount of protein and energy needed to optimize the use of nutrients, however, will depend on the pasture chemical composition and the crude protein/digestible organic matter (DOM) ratio, since ENU depends on the energy availability [11]. Therefore, supplementation must be preceded by the characterization of the quantity and quality of available forage, especially regarding the characteristics of carbohydrates and N compounds, to ensure the supply of nutrients that limit ruminal microbial activity [33].

2.3.1 Supplementation during dry season

Under conditions in Central Brazil, dry season is the most critical phase of grazing cattle production system. During this season, animals consume forage with low nutritional value, characterized by a high content of indigestible fiber and CP contents below critical level (7% CP), thus limiting its intake and, consequently, productive performance [27, 49]. Therefore, if there is no supplementation of cattle diet during this season, in order to supply the deficient nutrients of forage, there will be a reduction in weight gain or even negative performance, since the body nutrients are mobilized for maintenance, increasing the slaughter age, the fixed cost of the activity, and reducing livestock offtake rates [8].

According to Reis et al. [11], in the dry season, protein is the most limiting nutrient and, therefore, the one with the greatest need for supplementation, since it is a determinant in the capacity for fibrous substrates degradation by ruminal microorganisms and, consequently, in the passage rate and dry matter intake. In this sense, strategic supplementation during dry season involves the supply of protein, considering the ruminal events of digestion, fermentation, synthesis of N compounds and intake of low-quality forage. The live weight gains obtained through supplementation at this phase can be low, ensuring maintenance of animal weight, moderate (up to 300 g/animal/d), and even high (from 600 to 700 g/animal/d), enabling earlier slaughter of animals [8]. An advantageous alternative is the use of multiple supplements (protein and energy), which result in gains in the order of 150 to 300 g/animal/d with 0.5 to 2% BW and 700 to 1000 g/animal/d with 8 to 10% BW supplement.

2.3.2 Supplementation during rainy season

Although the rainy season is characterized by presenting edaphoclimatic conditions favorable to forage production, the way in which these conditions occur, associated to the management strategies adopted and the interactions between pasture quality and quantity and nutrient supply via supplement, can provide differences in the magnitude of responses to supplementation on animal performance and gain per area [48].

During this period, when forages are classified as medium to high-quality, with N compounds above the minimum recommended (7% CP) for full activity of bacteria using structural carbohydrates and with levels of rumen ammonia ($N\text{-}NH_3$) above 5 mg/dL, the objective of supplementation associated with grazing management strategies that maximize the production of grazing stratum, is to prevent deleterious effects in the use of potentially digestible NDF (pdNDF) in forage [49, 50]. According to Huhtanen et al. [50], pdNDF is a nutritionally more adequate entity for evaluating forage quality and corresponds to the portion of NDF that is potentially digested by ruminal microorganisms, and the digested amount is related to the retention time in the fermentation compartments, being short to complete the digestion of all the ingested pdNDF.

According to Santos et al. [51], values of average daily gain (ADG) above 800 g during the rainy season are hardly reached by cattle kept in tropical pastures without the use of supplementation with concentrate. Despite the high cost of the additional gains inherent to the concentrate in this period (100 to 200 g/animal/day), this can result in a considerable reduction in finishing phase time, on pasture or feedlot, with possible economic returns [6, 33, 36, 52].

2.3.3 Energy supplementation

The main objective of grazing cattle supplementation is to increase the intake of energy and nutrients relative to those found in exclusive pasture diets [27]. When forage and easily fermentable carbohydrates are provided, fibrolytic microorganisms must compete with non-fibrous carbohydrate (NFC) for substrates such as NH_3, peptides, sulfur, and branched-chain carbon skeletons for their growth. An adequate supplementation strategy would be to maximize the use of forage by optimizing its digestion, increasing the passage rate of indigestible residue, and consequently increasing the intake of TDN [9].

According to Poppi and McLennan [26], high weight gains depend mainly on the supply of amino acids and energy transported to bovine tissues, a condition that is rare in animals under exclusive grazing. In this context, the same authors reported that energy supply can be an effective strategy to provide extra protein to the animal, as it allows NH_3, which is usually lost in urine, feces, or saliva, to be captured and incorporated into microbial protein. Microbial protein production, in turn, varies depending on the nature of the energy substrate supplied, such as starch, soluble fiber, pectin or sugars [53].

In intensive production systems, tropical grasses managed with high N doses (200 to 500 kg/N/ha) during the rainy season present about 40 to 50% of nitrogenous compound content in soluble form [54]. This fact, associated with the high content of structural carbohydrates with lower degradation rates, promotes a lack of synchrony between N and carbon skeletons arising from the degradation of carbohydrates in the rumen, disfavoring microbial protein synthesis and the efficiency of ruminal N-NH_3 utilization [26].

For Poppi and McLennan [26], this condition causes excessive losses of nitrogenous compounds in the ruminal environment in the NH_3 form, decreasing the microbial protein synthesis and generating a metabolizable protein (MP) deficit in relation to the requirements for high gains. Also, according to the researchers, maximum efficiency in microbial protein synthesis is reached when 160 g CP/kg DOM is observed, while values close to 210 g CP/kg DOM result in appreciable N loss.

According to Reis et al. [8], the main limitations for ruminal microbial growth would be related to the forage available for grazing, allowing low assimilation of available N in ruminal microbial protein, due to the high degradability of N compounds or lower carbohydrate degradation rate from fibrous forage. Thus, the supply of energy supplements with sources of rapid availability in the rumen can promote better animal performance by optimizing the microbial assimilation of N from N compounds with high degradability in the forage [45].

In a review by Reis et al. [11], the authors reported that during the rainy season, tropical grasses have DM digestibility between 55 and 65%, in addition to CP between 7.9 and 17.4% in their composition, which can result in different CP/DOM ratios. Assessing experiments conducted in the rainy season, it was observed that even in animals receiving only mineral salt, ruminal N-NH_3 values are above the critical level of 5 mg/dL of rumen fluid [30, 34]. However, only when the animals were supplemented, in the first 6 hours after supplementation, optimal levels of N-NH_3 were found in the rumen for maximum microbial growth, i.e., greater than 20 mg of N-NH_3/dL of ruminal fluid.

According to Leng [55], the inclusion of grains in roughage diets can reduce fiber digestibility, and this phenomenon is inherent to two effects that interfere in cellulolytic bacteria growth: a specific effect (drop in pH) and a non-specific (carbohydrate effect). In ruminants raised on tropical pastures, the variation in ruminal pH as a function of dietary supplementation seems to be relatively small, not affecting growth of bacteria that use fibrous carbohydrates. In this sense, the availability of soluble carbohydrates is responsible for the depression of fiber digestibility, as reported by Rooke et al. [56] and Huhtanen [57], reflecting the high effectiveness of long fibers that act in the maintenance of ruminal conditions [58].

The goal of a supplementation program for grazing animals is, therefore, to satisfy their requirements through an interactive and associative action between the basal forage and the supplemental sources. Thus, it is possible to enhance the positive associative effects and minimize negative interactions, in order to increase intake and optimize forage use, and not only the direct meeting of animal requirements via supplement [27].

2.3.4 Protein supplementation

Protein is the main limitation in cattle production systems on tropical pasture both in the dry and rainy seasons, especially when the pastures have low nutritive value [59]. At that time, although some tropical grasses have CP levels that meet the animal's nutritional requirements, part of this protein may be unavailable to the action of ruminal microorganisms, as it is linked to fibrous fraction [8]. Therefore, the formulation of a protein or protein-energy supplement for grazing cattle must consider the protein fraction available of forage, to provide enough N to use the energy substrates contained in the plant, such as digestible cellulose and hemicellulose [33].

The additional supply of N for animals consuming low nutritive value forage favors the growth of fibrolytic bacteria, increases the digestibility and microbial protein synthesis and, thus, allows to increase the voluntary intake of forage and improve the energy balance of the grazing animal [60]. The success of this supplementation strategy is associated to characteristics of pdNDF fraction, which will be the main source of energy to meet the demand of microorganisms [11]. Once the N requirements for the maintenance of ruminal microorganisms are met, the supplement can provide protein and energy for additional gains, according to the desired performance [60].

According to Pathak [61], cattle need two types of protein: rumen degradable protein (RDP), which is necessary to meet the requirements of ruminal microorganisms, and rumen undegraded protein (RUP), to meet the requirements of animals. In this scenario, dietary protein acts as a source of MP for ruminants, which in turn corresponds to the sum of the microbial protein synthesized from the RDP, with the RUP absorbed in the intestine.

Microbial protein synthesis depends on adequate sources of N and carbohydrates. In this sense, Rodríguez et al. [62] report that the structure of dietary proteins defines their degradation in the rumen and the contribution to available N to microorganisms. Ammonia is the main source of N in rumen microorganisms, but the availability of amino acids, peptides, and both increase the growth of cellulolytic and amylolytic bacteria [63], mainly due to direct incorporation into microbial protein or increased availability of carbon skeletons that can be used as an energy source or in the synthesis of microbial amino acids [64].

In mixed forage and concentrate diets, microbial protein synthesis can be increased due to better synchronization of nutrient release, adequate ruminal environment for maintenance of different species of microorganisms, increased amounts and types of substrates, higher nutrient intake and, consequently, an increase in the rate of passage of solids and liquids [65]. While forages can supply N as highly degradable protein or non-protein nitrogen (NPN), concentrates can supply N primarily as peptides and/or amino acids needed for microbial protein synthesis [26]. According to Pathak [61], efficiency tends to increase when readily fermentable carbohydrate is supplemented in less than 30% of the total diet but decreases when the level of supplementation is greater than 70%.

In pasture systems, even during rainy season, the synchronism between protein and energy in the rumen is rarely achieved, due to variations in forage quality and different rates of substrate utilization [7]. However, urea recycling is an important ruminant mechanism, capable of ensuring adequate levels of N-NH_3 in the rumen throughout the day, however when there is excess protein in the diet, there may be losses of N to the environment [9]. In this sense, the great challenge in choosing the sources and amount of CP in the supplement is to equate its use according to energy availability, ensuring adequate levels of N-NH_3 and minimizing losses in feces and urine [9].

Protein supplements can be composed by two protein sources: true protein and NPN. True protein sources have different RDP contents, such as cottonseed meal and corn gluten, which have about 65 and 18% RDP in their composition, respectively [66].

Non-protein nitrogen sources are completely soluble in the rumen and used by ruminal bacteria for microbial protein synthesis, and its use is common, mainly due to its lower cost, when compared to other conventional protein source, such as soybean meal [67]. According to Araújo et al. [68], the main source of NPN used in Brazil is urea, which has become an advantageous alternative by its easy availability in the market, high concentration of N in its composition and low unit cost. Additionally, urea is a source of N-NH_3 for fibrolytic microorganisms and, because of its low acceptability, it can be used as a controlling agent for supplement intake by animals. However, it is essential to respect the limits of urea inclusion in the diet, to avoid causing poisoning in animals and high N loss in urine. For more efficient use of nutrients, urea should be mixed with energy components rich in non-fibrous carbohydrates, true protein, and sulfur.

In pasture production systems, it is necessary to optimize the use of nutrients and forage digestibility to maximize weight gain, even though the supplement promotes direct input of nutrients required by animal [66]. In this scenario, protein supplementation can increase forage intake due to the supply of N-NH_3 to ruminal microorganisms, and a consequent increase in energy intake, responsible for the increase in animal performance. However, the intensity of the response to a protein supplement will depend on pasture availability and quality [33].

2.4 Non-edible feed

In animal nutrition, corn is the main ingredient in energy supplements, and contains around 72% starch, 9% CP, low fiber content, in addition to being the largest source of metabolizable energy (ME) among cereals [69]. However, corn is an ingredient traditionally consumed by humans and monogastric animals which, in the context of system sustainability, generates competition between livestock and society [70]. Likewise, cottonseed meal and soybean meal are the most conventionally used protein ingredients in animal feed, due to the high CP content, which varies between 30 and 50%, and RUP, which contributes to increase the protein flow to the intestine [71–73]. Despite being important protein sources, they are costly ingredients that increase the production costs of beef cattle systems.

In the search for alternative feed not consumed by humans and for less costly ingredients in cattle nutrition, agroindustry co-products have gained prominence in the market and in research, especially in Brazil.

2.4.1 Citrus pulp

The orange juice and other citrus fruit industry, whose production leadership is in Brazil, generates bagasse or citrus pulp as a co-product, which comprises between 45 and 58% of the total fruit, consisting of peels, membranes, vesicles, and seeds of orange or another citrus. Nutritionally, it is characterized as an intermediate product between roughage and concentrates, rich in pectin, cellulose, and hemicellulose polysaccharides [74, 75].

Citrus pulp has been widely used to replace corn, presenting in its composition 85–90% of the energy value of this ingredient [76], in addition to having little or no negative effect on ruminal fermentation compared to starch-rich diets [74] .

In general, the pulp is characterized by high DM digestibility, high soluble fiber content, high soluble carbohydrate content and highly digestible cell wall [77]. In its chemical composition, citrus pulp has approximately 89–90% DM; 6–11% CP; 2–12% of ether extract (EE), this value depending on whether or not the oils are extracted during processing; 6% mineral matter (MM), 57–74% non-nitrogen extract (NNE); 7–8% crude fiber; 25–41% NDF; 14% of acid detergent fiber (ADF); 1% lignin, 0.2% starch, 22–25% pectin; 3.88 mg vitamin C/100 g by-product, 1.6–1.8% calcium and low phosphorus content (0.08–0.75%) [74, 78, 79].

Pectin consists of a structural carbohydrate, a component of the soluble fiber fraction, which in turn is a polymer of galacturonic acid [80]. According to Muller and Prado [77], co-products with a high concentration of pectin have great potential for use in ruminant nutrition, as it presents high energy density, in addition to favorable fermentation, without the production of lactic acid, which maintains adequate conditions for ruminal functioning.

Because it contains an extremely low starch content, citrus pulp can favor ruminal pH, preventing a sharp decrease during digestion, which can cause metabolic disturbances, in addition to providing maximum cellulolytic activity and a higher acetate:propionate ratio [64, 81–85].

In a study conducted by Oliveira et al. [34] evaluating three supplements, one mineral, one corn-based protein-energy supplement and the other based on citrus pulp, the authors concluded that citrus pulp as an energy source in supplements provided at 0.3% of body weight (BW) can be used in the supplementation of Nellore bulls during the rainy season, without compromising forage intake and fiber digestibility, improving ruminal microbial efficiency.

2.4.2 Dried distiller's grain (DDG)

Protein ingredients in the diet are usually considered the costliest. Thus, the search for alternatives that reduce production costs and even that do not generate competition with food consumed by humans in livestock systems has been increasingly intensified.

An alternative protein ingredient is dried distillers' grain with soluble (DDGs), a co-product of ethanol from corn or sorghum production, which has been gaining attention in animal nutrition for meeting the energy and protein demands of diets in pasture or feedlot systems [71]. In Brazil, however, most industries produce DDG without soluble, resulting from dry milling of corn processing for ethanol production [66]. DDG is typically characterized by its high protein content with low ruminal degradation, presenting between 50 and 62% of RUP in its composition, responsible for the greater supply of MP to the ruminant [86]. Comparatively, the RUP content of DDG is higher than that of cotton and soybean meal, 50 and 20%, respectively [87].

Chemical composition of DDG, however, varies depending on the type, variety and quality of grains, soil conditions, fertilization, irrigation, production and harvesting methods, in addition to factors related to processing in distilleries [88]. Tjardes & Wright [89] demonstrate variations in the nutritional characteristics of DDGs, ranging from 88 to 90% in DM content, 25 to 32% of CP, 43 to 53% in RDP, 47 to 57% in RUP, 39 to 45% of NDF, 8.8 to 12.4% of lipids and 85 to 90% of TDN in studies conducted with beef cattle. Furthermore, the co-product contains highly fermentable fiber and low starch content, which reduces the risk of acidosis in cattle consuming a high-grain diet, improving rumen health, in addition to being a source of minerals [90]. According to Fonseca et al. [86], in Brazil, the DDG produced by most companies does not have the reconstitution of the soluble fraction, presenting lower values of EE and non-fibrous carbohydrates.

In a study of Buckner et al. [91], the authors tested the inclusion of up to 40% of DDGs in the total DM diet and observed that the inclusion of the co-product resulted in higher ADG compared to the control diet. Other studies that evaluated the use of corn DDG at levels of 0; 50 and 100% replacement for conventional protein sources (cotton meal and soybean meal) reported that DDG can 100% replace the protein source during the rearing phase on tropical pastures without any adverse effects on ADG, enteric CH_4 emissions or N excretion [66, 92]. Furthermore, Hoffmann et al. [93] reported that the use of DDG does not affect animal performance finished in pasture or conventional feedlot, emphasizing that it is a viable alternative to replace conventional supplements in a tropical environment.

However, although DDG has the potential to replace conventional protein sources, its inclusion is limited mainly due to seasonal availability. In addition, unlike Brazil, countries such as the United States in some plants, use sulfuric acid for acidic starch hydrolysis during the processing of DDGs and for cleaning equipment, the excess of which can cause negative environmental impacts and even on the carcass quality [94, 95].

Other alternatives of agroindustry co-products that have been used in ruminant supplementation involve corn gluten, glycerin, and peanut crop residues, such as skin and husks.

2.5 Feed additives

In recent decades, the excessive use of antibiotics in animal production has resulted in a considerable increase in resistant bacteria, making it difficult to treat infectious animal diseases and compromising food safety [22]. These compounds are traditionally known as additives, which are defined as "substances intentionally added to feed, with the purpose of preserving, intensifying or modifying its properties, as long as it does not harm its nutritive value, such as antibiotics, dyes, preservatives, antioxidants among others" [96]. In general, additives are used to increase feed efficiency and animal performance, and are divided into different types, including ionophores, antimicrobials/antibiotics, microbial additives, organic acids, and plant extracts such as tannins, saponins and essential oils [97].

Ionophores are the most researched additives in ruminant diets, especially sodium monensin, and its use started in 1976 in beef cattle diets in the United States [98]. The action of ionophores in the rumen occurs through changes in the microbial population, selecting gram-negative bacteria that produce succinic and propionic acids or that ferment lactic acid, and inhibiting gram-positive bacteria that produce acetic, butyric, lactic and hydrogen (H_2) acids, precursor of enteric CH_4 production [98]. Due to this mechanism of action, the use of ionophores in ruminants can optimize energy metabolism, changing the proportion of volatile fatty acids (VFA) produced in the rumen and reducing CH_4 production, as well as improving N metabolism by ruminal microorganisms, decreasing the absorption of NH_3 and increasing the amount of protein that reaches the small intestine, in addition to reducing disorders arising from abnormal fermentation in the rumen, such as ruminal acidosis, bloat and coccidiosis [99].

Antibiotic additives have been used to promote growth for over 55 years, helping to reduce the cost of animal production. However, due to food safety, there are few antibiotics approved by agencies in different countries around the world [22]. The main products used include virginiamycin, bacitracin, flavomycin and tyrosine. In general, antibiotics act directly on rumen metabolism, as they modify the microbial rumen population to optimize ruminal fermentation and nutrient conservation, promoting antibacterial activity on gram-positive bacteria, activity against fungi and protozoa. Furthermore, antibiotics modify the ruminal digestibility of feed, reduce N degradation and enteric CH_4 production, and can control subclinical diseases by suppressing infectious bacteria [100].

Microbial additives are composed of live cells of microorganisms and/or their metabolites, including yeasts, fibrolytic enzymes and probiotics, especially *Aspergillus orizae, Sacchariomyces cerevisae* and *Lactobacillus ssp*, and their use has increased because they are "natural" substances that promote growth to improve production efficiency in ruminants [101]. In general, microbial additives act in the production of antimicrobial compounds (acids, bacteriocins, antibiotics), prevent the establishment of unwanted microorganisms, reestablish the microflora of the digestive tract, and also improve immunity and stimulate animal growth [101].

Furthermore, the use of fibrolytic enzymes can stimulate endogenous ruminal activity and increase the rate and extent of forage digestion by ruminants, due to the improvement in the colonization of feed particles [102].

According to Carro & Ungerfeld [103], organic acids are an alternative to antibiotics and in ruminant nutrition, the most used as additives include malic, fumaric, aspartate, citric, succinic, and pyruvic. As they do not produce detectable residues in meat, the use of organic acids does not cause risks to food safety, however their cost is high. In the rumen, these additives can favor the use of lactate and prevent a sharp drop in pH, preventing ruminal acidosis, and reduce the production of enteric CH_4.

As an alternative to antibiotics, many plants and plant extracts have received attention for their ability to manipulate ruminal fermentation and animal metabolism, in order to increase performance and promote beneficial effects to the environment [13]. Natural compounds commonly used in ruminant nutrition include condensed tannins, saponins and essential oils.

Condensed tannins (CT) are complexes composed of polyphenols, found in tropical legumes and other C3 plants, which bind to proteins, metal ions and polysaccharides, such as starch, cellulose, and hemicellulose [104]. When they exceed 6% of DM in the diet, CT are considered antinutritional factors because they reduce intake, fiber digestibility and animal performance, however in adequate doses (2–4% DM), CT can promote beneficial effects, especially in the regarding GHG emissions by ruminants [105]. These compounds can reduce protein degradation in the rumen and reduce NH_3 concentration along with less urinary N excretion [106]. Besides, CT can also reduce fiber fermentation in the rumen, which consequently reduces H_2 and acetate formation, in addition to inhibiting the growth of methanogenic microorganisms, thus reducing the production of enteric CH_4 [106, 107].

Saponins, in turn, are glycosides naturally present in some plants, such as *Medicago sativa* (alfafa) and *B. decumbens* and are used in animal nutrition as growth inhibitors of ruminal protozoa and modulators of ruminal fermentation in cattle [108]. Essential oils, on the other hand, comprise secondary metabolites of some plants, responsible for their odor and color, and are obtained by vaporization or distillation in water. According to Stevanović et al. [109], among the main essential oils, the most used are thymol present in thyme (*Thymus vulgaris*), oregano (*Origanum vulgaris*), limonene extracted from citrus pulp and guaiacol extracted from guaiac resin or clove oil from India. As a mechanism of action, these oils reduce the rate of deamination of amino acids, the rate of NH_3 production, with an increase in the ruminal escape of N into the intestine. Furthermore, it can increase the concentration of total VFA without affecting other fermentation parameters and even inhibit methanogenesis.

In the context of organic additives, the Fator P (Premix®, Patrocinio Paulista, Brazil) was designed and developed using 100% natural and national technology, being formed by a complex combination of amino acids, probiotics, and essential fatty acids, such as omega 3 and omega 6, in addition to organic minerals and surfactants. The use of this additive in the diet of ruminants can improve fiber digestion, ruminal metabolism, nutrient absorption and, thus, animal performance, in addition to meeting new market trends, associating sustainability and profitability.

Several metabolic studies conducted using the Fator P in ruminant diet demonstrated greater stability and performance of animal metabolism, through better intake and absorption of fibrous feed and, mainly, in the energy availability from diet, which resulted in a 20% increase in weight gain [110–112]. Furthermore, the additive promotes improvements in carcass quality and milk composition, can benefit the female reproduction and the immune system, thus reducing costs with sanitary management. In the context of sustainability, the Fator P optimizes the dynamics of ruminal microorganisms which, associated with greater stability in ruminal fermentation, can reduce GHG emissions per arroba produced by up to 36%, in addition to not causing microbial resistance, and can be used without restrictions, as opposed to conventional additives [112].

The use of these organic additives, therefore, can help to fully exploit the genetic potential of animals and pastures and improve the efficiency of use, in addition to reducing environmental damage, especially with lower emissions of greenhouse gases. In a study evaluating the use of this additive, Leite et al. [113] reported that it increased DM intake of the animals during the initial phase in a feedlot system and did not change the performance, when compared to the conventional additive, monensin.

3. Final considerations

Although livestock is considered the villain of global warming, grazing and nutritional management strategies are essential to mitigate GHG emissions. Proper grazing management results in forage with a higher nutritive value, allowing for more efficient use of nutrients, which increases animal performance. The intensification of pasture use implies the adoption of diet supplementation at different times of the year, aiming to maximize the productive animal performance. Supplementation of beef cattle during rearing in rainy season is an effective strategy to intensify the system due to the period of efficient animal gain and pasture quality. The use of alternative additives to antibiotics can promote better productive responses, in addition to reducing enteric CH_4 production and N_2O emission by excreta. However, when adopting pasture management and supplementation techniques, it is necessary to assess the economic and environmental impacts.

Acknowledgements

Financial support was provided by Premix® Company.

Conflict of interest

The authors declare no conflict of interest.

Notes/thanks/other declarations

The authors thank the members of UnespFor (Unesp Jaboticabal/SP Forage Team).

Author details

Andressa Scholz Berça[1*], Eliéder Prates Romanzini[1], Abmael da Silva Cardoso[1], Luís Eduardo Ferreira[2], André Pastori D'Aurea[2], Lauriston Bertelli Fernandes[2] and Ricardo Andrade Reis[1]

1 São Paulo State University, Jaboticabal, São Paulo, Brazil

2 Premix Company, Ribeirão Preto, São Paulo, Brazil

*Address all correspondence to: dessaberca@yahoo.com.br

References

[1] McManus C, Barcellos JO, Formenton BK, Hermuche PM, Carvalho OA, Guimarães R, Gianezini M, Dias EA, Lampert Vd, Zago D, Neto JB. Dynamics of Cattle Production in Brazil. Plos One. 2016;11(1):e0147138. DOI: 10.1371/journal.pone.0147138

[2] Abiec - Associação Brasileira das Indústrias Exportadoras de Carnes. Beef Report: Perfil da Pecuária no Brasil [Internet]. 2021. Available from: http://abiec.com.br/publicacoes/beef-report-2021/. [Accessed: 2021-07-20].

[3] Dubeux Jr, JCB, Sollenberger JCB, Muir JP, Tedeschi LO, Dos Santos MV, da Cunha MV, Dilorenzo N. Sustainable intensification of livestock production on pastures. Archivos Latinoamericanos de Producción Animal. 2017; 25:3-4

[4] Cardoso AS, Berndt A, Leytem BJR, Alves IDN, DeCarvalho LH, De Barros Soares S, Urquiaga, Boddey RM. Impact of the intensification of beef production in Brazil on greenhouse gas emissions and land use. Agricultural Systems. 2016; 143:86-92. DOI: 10.1016/j.agsy.2015.12.007

[5] Cardoso AS, Barbero RP, Romanzini EP, Teobaldo RW, Ongaratto F, Fernandes MHMR, Ruggieri AC, Reis RA. Intensification: A key strategy to achieve great animal and environmental beef cattle production sustainability in Brachiaria grasslands. Sustainability. 2020; 12:6656. DOI: 10.3390/su12166656

[6] Delevatti LM, Romanzini EP, Koscheck JFW, Araujo TLR, Renesto DM, Ferrari AC, Barbero RP, Mullinikis JT, Reis RA. Forage management intensification and supplementation strategy: Intake and metabolic parameters on beef cattle production. Animal Feed Science and Technology. 2019;247:74-82. DOI: 10.1016/j.anifeedsci.2018.11.004

[7] De Jesus FLF, Sanches AC, De Souza DP, Mendonça FC, Gomes EP, Santos RC, Da Silva JLB. Seasonality of biomass production of irrigated Mombaça 'Guinea grass'. Acta Agriculturae Scandinavica, Soil e Plant Science. 2021;1-9. DOI: 10.1080/09064710.2020.1863456

[8] Reis RR, Ruggieri AC, Oliveira AA, Azenha MV, Casagrande DR. Suplementação como estratégia de produção de carne de qualidade em pastagens tropicais. Revista Brasileira de Saúde e Produção Animal. 2012;642-655. ISSN 1519 9940.

[9] Poppi DP, Quigley SP, Silva TACCD, McLennan SR. Challenges of beef cattle production from tropical pastures. Revista Brasileira de Zootecnia. 2018;47:1-9. DOI: 10.1590/rbz472016041

[10] Valadares Filho S, Silva FAZ, Benedeti PDB, Paulino MF, Chizzotti ML. Nutrient requirements of beef cattle in tropical climates. EAAP Scientific Series. 2019. DOI: 10.3920/978-90-8686-891-9

[11] Reis RA, Ruggieri AC, Casagrande DR, Páscoa AG. Suplementação da dieta de bovinos de corte como estratégia do manejo das pastagens. Revista Brasileira de Zootecnia. 2019;38:147-159. DOI: 10.1590/S1516-35982009001300016

[12] Peyrald JL. The role of grassland-based production system for sustainable protein production. In: Proceedings of the Annual meeting of the Brazilian society of Animal Science; July 2017; Foz do Iguaçu, Brazil. 2017. p.243-255. hal-01591147

[13] Hart KJ, Yáñez-Ruiz DR, Duval SM, McEwan NR, Newbold CJ. Plant extracts

to manipulate rumen fermentation. Animal Feed Science and Technology. 2008;147:8-35. DOI: 10.1016/j.anifeedsci.2007.09.007

[14] Herrero M, Havlík P, Valin H, Notenbaert A, Rufino MC, Thornton PK, Obersteiner M. Biomass use, production, feed efficiencies, and greenhouse gas emissions from global livestock systems. In: Proceedings of the National Academy of Sciences; December 2013; Cambridge. 2013. p. 20888-20893. DOI: 10.1073/pnas.1308149110

[15] FAO – Food and Agriculture Organization of the United Nations. Tackling climate change through livestock. A global assessment of emissions and mitigation opportunities. Rome, FAO, 115p., 2013.

[16] Berça AS, Cardoso AS, Longhini VZ, Tedeschi LO, Boddey RM, Berndt A, Reis RA, Ruggieri AC. Methane production and nitrogen balance of dairy heifers grazing palisade grass cv. Marandu alone or with forage peanut. Journal of Animal Science. 2019;97: 4625-4634. DOI: 10.1093/jas/skz310

[17] IPCC - Intergovernmental Panel on Climate Change. 2019 Refinement to the 2006 IPCC Guidelines for National Greenhouse Gas Inventories [Internet]. 2019. Available from: https://www.ipcc-nggip.iges.or.jp/public/2019rf/index.html [Accessed 2021-05-15].

[18] GLEAM - Global Livestock Environmental Assessment Model – GLEAM. 2019. Available from: http://www.fao.org/gleam/en/[Accessed 2021-05-15].

[19] Longhini VZ, Cardoso AS, Berça AS, Boddey RM, Reis RA, Dubeux JC, Ruggieri AC. Nitrogen supply and Rainfall affect Ammonia emissions from Dairy Cattle excreta and Urea applied on warm-climate pastures. Journal of Environmental Quality. 2020; 49:1453-1466. DOI: 10.1002/jeq2.20167

[20] Xu R, Tian H, Pan S, Prior AS, Feng Y, Batchelor WD, Yang J. Global ammonia emissions from synthetic nitrogen fertilizer applications in agricultural systems: Empirical and process-based estimates and uncertainty. Global Change Biology. 2019;25:314-326. DOI:10.1111/gcb.14499

[21] Foley JA, Ramankutty N, Brauman KA, Cassidy ES, Gerber JS, Johnston M, Zaks DP. Solutions for a cultivated planet. Nature. 2011;478:337-342. DOI: 10.1038/nature10452

[22] Tedeschi LO, Callaway TR, Muir JP, Anderson RC. Potential environmental benefits of feed additives and other strategies for ruminant production. Revista Brasileira de Zootecnia. 2011;40:291-309.

[23] Hatfield RD, Kalscheur KF. Carbohydrate and Protein Nutritional Chemistry of Forages. Forages: The Science of Grassland Agriculture. 2020;2:595-607. DOI: 10.1002/9781119436669.ch33

[24] Hristov AN, Ott T, Tricarico J, Rotz A, Waghorn G, Adesogan A, Firkins JL. Special topics - Mitigation of methane and nitrous oxide emissions from animal operations: III. A review of animal management mitigation options. Journal of Animal Science. 2013;11:5095-5113. DOI: 10.2527/jas.2013-6585

[25] Ruggieri AC, Cardoso AS, Ongaratto F, Casagrande DR, Barbero RP, Brito LF, Azenha MV, Oliveira AA, Koscheck JHW, Reis RA. Grazing Intensity Impacts on Herbage Mass, Sward Structure, Greenhouse Gas Emissions, and Animal Performance: Analysis of Brachiaria Pastureland. Agronomy. 2020;11:1750. DOI: 10.3390/agronomy10111750

[26] Poppi DP, McLennan SR. Protein and energy utilization by ruminants at pasture. Journal of Animal Science. 1995;73:278-290.

[27] Paulino MF, Figueiredo DD, Moraes EHBK, Porto MO, Sales MF, Acedo TS, Valadares Filho SDC. Suplementação de bovinos em pastagens: uma visão sistêmica. Simpósio de produção de gado de corte. 2004;4:93-144.

[28] Sollenberger LE, Newman YC, Macoon B. Pasture Design and Grazing Management. Forages: The Science of Grassland Agriculture. 2020;2:803-814. DOI: 10.1002/9781119436669.ch44

[29] Pereira JC, Gomes FK, Oliveira MD, Lara MA, Bernardes TF, Casagrande DR. Defoliation management affects morphogenetic and structural characteristics of mixed pastures of brachiaria grass and forage peanut. African Journal of Range e Forage Science. 2017;34:13-19. DOI: 10.2989/10220119.2017.1315960

[30] Casagrande DR, Ruggieri AC, Moretti MH, Berchielli TT, Vieira BR, Roth APTP, Reis RA. Sward canopy structure and performance of beef heifers under supplementation in *Brachiaria brizantha* cv. Marandu pastures maintained with three grazing intensities in a continuous stocking system. Revista Brasileira de Zootecnia. 2011;40:2074-2082. DOI: 10.1590/S1516-35982011001000002

[31] Baldissera TC, Pontes LS, Giostri AF, Barro RS, Lustosa SBC, De Moraes A, De Faccio Carvalho PC. Sward structure and relationship between canopy height and light interception for tropical C4 grasses growing under trees. Crop and Pasture Science. 2016;67:1199-1207. DOI: 10.1071/CP16067

[32] Azenha MV. Morfogênese e dinâmica do perfilhamento do capim-marandu submetido a alturas de pastejo em lotação contínua com e sem suplementação [dissertation]. Jaboticabal: Faculdade de Ciências Agrárias e Veterinária – UNESP; 2010.

[33] Barbero RP, Malheiros EB, Araújo TLR, Nave RLG, Mullinikis JT, Berchielli TT, Ruggieri AC, Reis RA. Combining Marandu grass grazing height and supplementation level to optimize growth and productivity of yearling bulls. Animal Feed Science and Technology. 2015;209:110-118. DOI: 10.1016/j.anifeedsci.2015.09.010

[34] Oliveira AP, Casagrande DR, Bertipaglia LMA, Barbero RP, Berchielli TT, Ruggieri AC, Reis RA. Supplementation for beef cattle on Marandu grass pastures with different herbage allowances. Animal Production Science. 2016;56:123-129. DOI: 10.1071/AN14636

[35] Vieira BR, Azenha MV, Casagrande DR, Costa DFA, Ruggieri AC, Berchielli TT, Reis RA. Ingestive behavior of supplemented Nellore heifers grazing palisadegrass pastures managed with different sward heights. Journal of Animal Science. 2017;4:696-704. DOI: 10.1111/asj.12696

[36] Koscheck FJW, Romanzini EP, Barbero RP, Delevatti LM, Ferrari AC, Mullininks JT, Mousquer CJ, Berchielli TT, Reis RA. How do animal performance and methane emissions vary with forage management intensification and supplementation?. Animal Production Science. 2020;1:1201-1209. DOI: 10.1071/AN18712

[37] Barbero RP, Malheiros EB, Aguilar NM, Romanzini EP, Ferrari AC, Nave RLG, Mullinks JT, Reis RA. Supplementation level increasing dry matter intake of beef cattle grazing low herbage height. Journal of Applied Animal Research. 2020;48:28-33. DOI: 10.1080/09712119.2020.1715985

[38] Delevatti LM, Cardoso AS, Barbero RP, Leite RG, Romanzini EP, Ruggieri AC, Reis RA. Effect of nitrogen application rate on yield, forage quality, and animal performance in a tropical pasture. Scientific Reports. 2019;9:1-9. DOI: 10.1038/s41598-019-44138-x

[39] Trindade JKD, Silv SCD, Souza Júnior SJD, Giacomini AA, Zeferino CV, Guarda VDA, Carvalho PCDF. Composição morfológica da forragem consumida por bovinos de corte durante o rebaixamento do capim-marandu submetido a estratégias de pastejo rotativo. Pesquisa Agropecuária Brasileira. 2007;6: 883-890. DOI: 10.1590/S0100-204X2007000600016

[40] Pedreira BC, Pedreira CGS, Da Silva SC. Estrutura do dossel e acúmulo de forragem de Brachiaria brizantha cultiva Xaraés em resposta a estratégias de pastejo. Pesquisa Agropecuária Brasileira. 2007;2:281-287. DOI: 10.1590/S0100-204X2007000200018

[41] Boddey RM, Macedo R, Tarré RM, Ferreira E, Oliveira OC, Rezende CP, Cantarutti RB, Pereira JM, Alves BJR, Urquiaga S. Nitrogen cycling in Brachiaria pastures: The key to understanding the process of pasture decline. Agriculture, Ecosystems e Environment. 2004;103:389-403. DOI: 10.1016/j.agee.2003.12.010

[42] Sollenberger L, Coleman SW, Vendramini JMB. A interação planta-herbívoros em pastagens. In: Reis RA, Bernardes TF, Siqueira GR, editors. Handbook of Forragicultura Ciência, Tecnologia e Gestão dos Recursos Forrageiros. 1st ed. Gráfica Multipress: Jaboticabal, Brazil; 2014. p. 69-80.

[43] Rezende AV, Lima JF, Rabelo CHS, Rabelo FHS, Nogueira DA, Carvalho M, Faria Jr CNA, Barbosa LA. Características morfofisiológicas da Brachiaria brizantha cv. Marandu em resposta à adubação fosfatada. Agrarian. 2011;4:335-343.

[44] Balsalobre MAA, Corsi M, Santos PM, Cárdenas RR. Composição química e fracionamento do nitrogênio e dos carboidratos do capim-tanzânia irrigado sob três níveis de resíduo pós-pastejo. Revista da Sociedade Brasileira de Zootecnia. 2003;32:519-528.

[45] Detmann E, Valente EE, Batista ED, Huhtanen P. An evaluation of the performance and efficiency of nitrogen utilization in cattle fed tropical grass pastures with supplementation. Livestock Science. 2014;165:141-153.

[46] Aboyage IA, Oba M, Castillo AR, Koenig KM, Iwaasa AD, Beauchemin KA. Effects of hydrolyzable tannin with or without condensed tannin on methane emissions, nitrogen use, and performance of beef cattle fed a high-forage diet. Journal of Animal Science. 2018;96:5276-5286. DOI: 10.1093/jas/sky352

[47] Goés RHT, Alves DD, Mancio AB, Zercoudakis JT. Efeito Associativo na suplementação de bovinos a pasto. Arquivo de Ciências Veterinária e Zoologia da UNIPAR. 2004;7:169-169.

[48] Reis RA, Barbero RP, Hoffmann A. Impactos da qualidade da forragem em sistemas de produção de bovinos de corte. Informe Agropecuário. 2016;292:36-53.

[49] Paulino MF, Detmann E, Valadares Filho SC. Suplementação animal em pasto: energética ou protéica? In: Proceedings of Simpósio sobre manejo estratégico da pastagem; Viçosa, Brazil; 2006. p.359-392.

[50] Huhtanen P, Sudekum KH, Nousiainen J, Shingfield KJ. Forage conservation, feeding value and milk quality. Grassland in a changing world. 2010;15:379-400.

[51] Santos FAP, Correia PS, Ramalho TR, Costa DFA. Sistemas intensivos de recria de bovinos com

suplementação em pastagens e confinamento. In: Proceedings of Simpósio sobre Bovinocultura de Corte: Requisitos de qualidade na bovinocultura de corte; Piracicaba, Brazil; 2007. p. 183-219.

[52] Romanzini EP, Barbero RP, Reis RA, Hadley D, Malheiros EB. Economic evaluation from beef cattle production industry with intensification in Brazil's tropical pastures. Tropical Animal Health and Production. 2020;52:2659-2666. DOI: 10.1007/s11250-020-02304-8

[53] Dewhurst RJ, Davies DR, Merry RJ. Microbial protein supply from the rumen. Animal Feed Science and Technology. 2000;85:1-21. DOI: 10.1016/S0377-8401(00)00139-5

[54] Johnson CR, Reiling BA, Mislevy P, Hall MB. Effects of nitrogen fertilization and harvest date on yield, digestibility, fiber, and protein fractions of tropical grasses. Journal of Animal Science. 2001;79:2439-2448. DOI: 10.2527/2001.7992439x

[55] Leng RA. Factors affecting the utilization of "poor-quality" forages by ruminants particularly under tropical conditions. Nutrition Research Review. 1990;3:277- 303. DOI: 10.1079/NRR19900016

[56] Rooke JA, Lee NH, Armstrong DG. The effects of intraruminal infusions of urea, casein, glucose syrup and a mixture of glucose syrup and casein on nitrogen digestion in the rumen of cattle receiving grass silage diets. British Journal of Nutrition. 1987;57:89-98. DOI: 10.1079/BJN19870012

[57] Huhtanen P. The effects of intraruminal infusions of sucrose and xylose on the nitrogen and fibre digestion in the rumen of cattle receiving diets of grass silage and barley. Agriculture and Food Science. 1987;59:101-120. DOI: 10.23986/afsci.72274

[58] Mertens DR. Regulation of forage intake. In: Fahey Jr, editor. Forage quality, evaluation and utilization. American Society of Agronomy: Madison; 1994. p.450-493.

[59] Costa DFA, Correia PS, Dorea JRR, De Souza J, De Souza Congio CF, Pires AV, Santos FAP. Strategic supplementation of growing cattle on tropical pastures improves nutrient use and animal performance, with fewer days required on the finishing phase. Animal Production Science. 2020;81:480-493. DOI: 10.1071/AN20005

[60] Reis WLS, Detmann E, Batista ED, Rufino LMA, Gomes DI, Bento CBP, Valadares Filho SC. Effects of ruminal and post-ruminal protein supplementation in cattle fed tropical forages on insoluble fiber degradation, activity of fibrolytic enzymes, and the ruminal microbial community profile. Animal Feed Science and Technology. 2016;218:1-16. DOI: 10.1016/j.anifeedsci.2016.05.001

[61] Pathak AK. Various factors affecting microbial protein synthesis in the rumen. Veterinary World. 2008;6:186.

[62] Rodriguez R, Sosa A, Rodriguez Y. Microbial protein synthesis in rumen and its importance to ruminants. Cuban Journal of Agricultural Science. 2007;41:287-294.

[63] Kozloski GV. Ruminants Biochemistry. 3rd ed. Santa Maria: UFSM; 2011. 216p. ISBN 9788573911503.

[64] Van Soest PJ. Nutritional ecology of the ruminant. 2nd ed. Cornell University; 1994. 476p.

[65] Gomes MJ, Hovell FD, Chen XB, Nengomasha EM, Fikremariam D. The effect of starch supplementation of straw on microbial protein supply in sheep. Animal Feed Science and Technology. 1994;49:277-286.

[66] Hoffmann A, Cardoso AS, Fonseca NVB, Romanzini EP, Siniscalchi D, Berndt A, Ruggieri AC, Reis RA. Effects of supplementation with corn distillers' dried grains on animal performance, nitrogen balance, and enteric CH_4 emissions of young Nellore bulls fed a high-tropical forage diet. Animal. 2021;15:100155. DOI: 10.1016/j.animal.2020.100155

[67] Tadele Y, Amha N. Use of different non protein nitrogen sources in ruminant nutrition: a review. Advances in Life Science and Technology. 2015;29:84-89.

[68] Araújo HPDO, Paula NFD, Martello HF, Teobaldo RW, Pereira LB, Mora LM, Antunes HCF. Urea and Tannin in multiple supplements: Ingestive behavior of grazing beef cattle. Acta Scientiarum. Animal Sciences. 2020;42. DOI: 10.4025/actascianimsci.v42i1.47607

[69] Loy DD, Lundy EL. Nutritional properties and feeding value of corn and its coproducts. In: Corn. AACC International Press; 2019. p. 633-659.

[70] Mottet A, Teillard F, Boettcher P, De' Besi G, Besbes B. Review: domestic herbivores and food security: current contribution, trends and challenges for a sustainable development. Animal. 2018;12:188-198. DOI: 10.1017/S1751731118002215

[71] Swiatkiewicz S, Arczewska-Wlosek A, Józefiak D. The use of cottonseed meal as a protein source for poultry: An updated review. World's Poultry Science Journal. 2016;72:473-484. DOI: 10.1017/S0043933916000258

[72] Paula EM, Broderick GA, Danes MAC, Lobos NE, Zanton GI, Faciola AP. Effects of replacing soybean meal with canola meal or treated canola meal on ruminal digestion, omasal nutrient flow, and performance in lactating dairy cows. Journal of Dairy Science. 2018;101:328-339. DOI: 10.3168/jds.2017-13392

[73] Hoffmann A, Cardoso AS, Fonseca NVB, Romanzini EP, Siniscalchi D, Berndt A, Ruggieri AC, Reis RA. Effects of supplementation with corn distillers' dried grains on animal performance, nitrogen balance, and enteric CH_4 emissions of young Nellore bulls fed a high-tropical forage diet. Animal. 2021;1:100155. DOI: 10.1016/j.animal.2020.100155

[74] Bampidis VA, Robinson PH. Citrus by-products as ruminant feeds: a review. Animal Feed Science and Technology. 2006;128:175-217. DOI: 10.1016/j.anifeedsci.2005.12.002

[75] Franzolin R, Franzolin MHT. População protozoários ciliados e degradabilidade ruminal em búfalos e bovinos zebuínos sob dieta à base de cana-de-açúcar. Revista Brasileira de Zootecnia. 2000;29:1853-1861. DOI: 10.1590/S1516-35982000000600034

[76] NRC - National Research Council. Nutrient Requirements of Beef Cattle. 7th ed. Washington, DC, USA: Natl. Acad. Press, 2000.

[77] Muller M, Prado IN. Metabolismo da pectina para produção de carne e leite em ruminantes. In: IN Prado, editor. Conceitos sobre a produção com qualidade de carne e leite. Maringá, Brazil: 2004. pp. 115-146.

[78] Oluremi OIA, Ojighen VO, Ejembi EH. The nutritive potentials of sweet orange (*Citrus sinensis*) rind in broiler production. International Journal of Poultry Science. 2006;5:613-617.

[79] Watanabe PH, Thomaz MC, Ruiz US, Santos VM, Masson GC, Fraga AL, Silva SZ. Carcass characteristics and meat quality of heavy swine fed different citrus pulp levels. Arquivo Brasileiro de Medicina

Veterinária e Zootecnia. 2010;62:921-929. DOI: 10.1590/S0102-09352010000400023

[80] Santos FAP, Carmo CDA, Bittar CMM, Pires AV, Pedroso AM, Pereira EM. Milho com diferentes graus de moagem em combinação com polpa cítrica peletizada ou casca de soja para vacas leiteiras no terço médio da lactação. Revista Brasileira de Zootecnia. 2007;36:1183-1191. DOI: 10.1590/S1516-35982007000500027

[81] Cullen AJ, Harmon DL, Nagaraja TG. In vitro fermentation of sugars, grains and by-product feeds in relation to initiation of ruminal lactate production. Journal of Dairy Science. 1986;69:2616-2623. DOI: 10.3168/jds.S0022-0302(86)80709-3

[82] Strobel HJ, Russell JB. Effect of pH and energy spilling on bacterial protein synthesis by carbohydrate limited cultures of mixed rumen bacteria. Journal of Dairy Science. 1986;69:2941-2953. DOI: 10.3168/jds.S0022-0302(86)80750-0

[83] Belyea RL, Steevens BJ, Restrepo RJ, Clubb AP. Variation in composition of by-product feeds. Journal of Dairy Science. 1989;72:2339-2345. DOI: 10.3168/jds.S0022-0302(89)79366-8

[84] Van Soest PJ, Robertson JB, Lewis BA. Methods of dietary fiber, neutral detergent fiber, and nonstarch polysaccharides in relation to animal nutrition. Journal of Dairy Science. 1991;74:3583-3597. DOI: 10.3168/jds.S0022-0302(91)78551-2

[85] Porcionato MAF, Berchielli TT, Franco GL. Avaliação dos parâmetros ruminais da polpa cítrica peletizada. 1-Degradação da MS e FDN. In: Proceedings of Reunião Anual da Sociedade Brasileira de Zootecnia. Viçosa: 2000. p. 347.

[86] Fonseca NVB, Cardoso AS, Hoffmann A, Leite RG, Ferrari AC, Fernandes MHMR, Reis RA. Characterization and effects of DDG on the intake and digestibility of finishing bulls in feedlots. Acta Scientiarum. 2020:43. DOI: 10.4025/actascianimsci.v43i1.51877

[87] Santos FAP, Pedroso AM. Suplementação proteica e energética para bovinos de corte em confinamento. In: Pires AV, editor. Bovinocultura de corte. Piracicaba: FEALQ, 2010. p. 257-280.

[88] Bottger C, Sudekum KH. European distillers dried grains with solubles (DDGS): Chemical composition and in vitro evaluation of feeding value for ruminants. Animal Feed Science and Technology. 2017;224:66-70. DOI: 10.1016/j.anifeedsci.2016.12.012

[89] Tjardes J, Wright C. Feeding corn distiller's co-products to beef cattle. Animal and Range Sciences. 2002:1-5.

[90] Freitas TB, Relling AE, Pedreira MS, Junior HAS, Felix TL. Effects of sodium hydroxide treatment of dried distillers' grains on digestibility, ruminal metabolism, and metabolic acidosis of feedlot steers1. Journal of Animal Science. 2016;94:709-717. DOI: 10.2527/jas.2015-9431

[91] Buckner CD, Mader TL, Erickson GE, Colgan SL, Mark DR, Karges KK, Bremer VR. Evaluation of dry distillers' grains plus solubles inclusion on performance and economics of finishing beef steers. The Professional Animal Scientist. 2008;24:404-410. DOI: 10.15232/S1080-7446(15)30884-6

[92] Ferrari AC. Aportes nutricionais na recria a pasto e sistemas na terminação de tourinhos Nelore: metabolismo, desempenho e qualidade da carne [thesis]. Jaboticabal: Faculdade de Ciências Agrárias e Veterinária - UNESP, 2019. 150p.

[93] Hoffmann A, Berça AS, Cardoso ADS, Fonseca NVB, Silva MLC, Leite RG, Ruggieri AC, Reis RA. Does the Effect of Replacing Cottonseed Meal with Dried Distiller's Grains on Nellore Bulls Finishing Phase Vary between Pasture and Feedlot?. Animals. 2021;11:85. DOI: 10.3390/ani11010085

[94] Smith WB, Banta JP, Foster JL, Redmon LA, Tedeschi LO, Rouquette FM. Impact of DDGS Supplementation of Cattle Grazing Bermudagrass on the Plant-Animal-Environment Nexus. Journal of Animal Science. 2016;95:62-63. DOI: 10.2527/ssasas2017.0127

[95] Council US Grains. A guide to distiller's dried grains with solubles (DDGS). 2013. Available from: http:// www. ddgs. umn. edu/prod/groups/ cfans/@ pub/@ cfans/@ ansci/ documents/ass et/cfans_asset_417244. pdf [Accessed 2021/06/25].

[96] Lanna DPD, Medeiros SR. Uso de aditivos na bovinocultura de corte. In: Santos FAP, Moura JC, Faria VP, editors. Requisitos de qualidade na bovinocultura de corte. Piracicaba: Fealq, 2007. p.297-324.

[97] Danieli B, Schogor ALB. Uso de aditivos na nutrição de ruminantes: revisão. Veterinária e Zootecnia. 2020;27:1-13. DOI: 10.35172/rvz.2020.v27.444

[98] Azzaz HH, Murad HA, Morsy TA. Utility of ionophores for ruminant animals: a review. Asian Journal of Animal Sciences. 2015;9:254-265. DOI: 10.3923/ajas.2015.254.265

[99] Tedeschi LO, Fox DG, Tylutki TP. Potential environmental benefits of ionophores in ruminant diets. Journal of environmental quality. 2003;32:1591-1602. DOI: 10.2134/jeq2003.1591

[100] McGrath J, Duval SM, Tamassia LF, Kindermann M, Stemmler RT, De Gouvea VN, Celi P. Nutritional strategies in ruminants: A lifetime approach. Research in Veterinary Science. 2018;116:28-39. DOI: 10.1016/j.rvsc.2017.09.011

[101] Arowolo MA, He J. Use of probiotics and botanical extracts to improve ruminant production in the tropics: A review. Animal Nutrition. 2018;4:241-249. DOI: 10.1016/j.aninu.2018.04.010

[102] Tirado-Gonzalez DN, Miranda-Romero LA, Ruíz-Flores A, Medina-Cuéllar SE, Ramírez-Valverde R, Tirado-Estrada G. Meta-analysis: effects of exogenous fibrolytic enzymes in ruminant diets. Journal of Applied Animal Research. 2018;46:771-783. DOI: 10.1080/09712119.2017.1399135

[103] Carro MD, Ungerfeld EM. Utilization of organic acids to manipulate ruminal fermentation and improve ruminant productivity. In: Rumen microbiology: from evolution to revolution. Springer, New Delhi, 2015. p. 177-197. DOI: 10.1007/978-81-322-2401-3_13

[104] Muir JP, Terrill T, Valencia E, Stuart W, Jones PD, Moskidis J, Wolfe R. The wide range of condensed tannins in Caribbean Basin plants and their applicability to ruminant production systems. In: Proceedings of Caribbean Food Crops Society Annual Meeting. St. Kitts and Nevi: Caribbean Food Crops Society, 2009. p.46-52. DOI: 10.22004/ag.econ.256353

[105] Martin C, Morgavi DP, Doreau M. Methane mitigation in ruminants: from microbes to the farm scale. Animal. 2009;4:351-365. DOI: 10.1017/S1751731109990620

[106] Patra AK, Saxena J. Exploitation of dietary tannins to improve rumen metabolism and ruminant nutrition. Journal of the Science of Food and

Agriculture. 2011;91:24-37. DOI: 10.1002/jsfa.4152

[107] Beauchemin KA, Kreuzer M, O'Mara F, McAllister TA. Nutritional management for enteric methane abatement: a review. Australian Journal of Experimental Agriculture. 2008;48:21-27. DOI: 10.1071/EA07199

[108] Silva NV, Costa RG, Freitas CRG, Galindo MCT, Silva RS. Alimentação de ovinos em regiões semiáridas do Brasil. Acta Veterinaria Brasilica. 2010;4:233-241. DOI: 10.21708/avb.2010.4.4.1906

[109] Stevanovic ZD, Bosnjak-Neumuller J, Pajic-Lijakovic I, Raj J, Vasiljevic M. Essential oils as feed additives—future perspectives. Molecules. 2018;23:1717. DOI: 10.3390/molecules23071717

[110] Fernandes LB, D'Áurea AP, Ferreira LE. Sustainable and efficient production of growing steers in the tropical pastures. In: Proceedings of 10th International Symposium on the Nutrition of Herbivores; 2-6 September 2018; Clermont, France; 2018. p.470

[111] D'Aurea AP, Fernandes LB, Ferreira LE, Pinto LD, Shiozaki FA. Welfare and Sustainability in Beef Cattle Production on Tropical Pasture. In: Procceedings of International Conference on Animal Welfare, Development, Conservation and Control; 22-23 April 2019; Newyork, USA; 2019. 13:4.

[112] Oliveira AP, Romanzini EP, Leite RG, Delevatti LM, Fernandes LB, D'Áurea AP, Reis RA. Feeding behavior during adaptation phase of beef cattle in feedlot reducing the use of conventional growth promoters. In: EAAP Scientific Series. Wageningen Academic Publishers, 2019. p.2538-2547. DOI: 10.3920/978-90-8686-891-9

[113] Leite RG, Romanzini EP, Delevatti LM, Hoffmann A, Ferrari AC, D'Áurea AP, Fernandes LB, Oliveira AP, Reis RA. Organic additives used in beef cattle feedlot: Effects on metabolic parameters and animal performance. Journal of Animal Science. 2019;00:1-9. DOI: 10.1111/asj.13183

Chapter 3

Potential Utilization of Insect Meal as Livestock Feed

Sipho Moyo and Busani Moyo

Abstract

Globally, the utilization of alternative protein sources in livestock feed has been extensively deliberated and established to be the best novel approach. Extensive research indicated that insects provide good opportunities as a sustainable, high quality, and low-cost component of animal feed. The use of insects in animal diet sounds to be the prospective opportunity leading to sustainability of animal feeds and meet the intensifying worldwide plea for livestock products. The value of these protein sources has, however, increased due to limited production, competition between humans and animals. The use of insects for feeding farmed animals represents a promising alternative because of the nutritional properties of insects and the possible environmental benefits, given the sustainability of this type of farming. Yet little has been documented about the nutrient composition of various insect meals, the impact of insect meal in the animal feed industry, safety, and attitude and willingness of farmers to accept insect-based animal feed and food. Therefore, this chapter seeks to document the potential utilization of insect meal as livestock feed.

Keywords: insect meal, safety, acceptance, chitin, benefits

1. Introduction

The Food and Agriculture Organization (FAO) emphasized the importance of alternatives to conventional animal feed due to limited amounts [1]. Currently, the core protein sources in monogastric animal diets are fishmeal, processed animal protein, milk by-product, soybean meal (SBM), rapeseed meal, and canola meal. The value of these protein sources has, however, increased due to limited production, competition between humans and animals [2]. In addition, Makkar et al. [3] stated that insects are good novel protein sources at a low-cost, with regard to their high nutritional value and low breeding space requirements. They are recommended as high quality, effective, ecological substitute sources of protein. More so, protein-enriched insects are another alternative reckoned to reduce the price of protein supplements in poultry diets. In addition, according to [4] insect components such as chitin, lauric acid, and antimicrobial peptides promote chicken health. Also, take into consideration that these insects can be utilized as a dried or fresh state in poultry diets [5]. Recently, scientists have started to study insects as state-of-the-art feed constituents for aquaculture [6, 7] and poultry [8, 9]. However, this chapter focuses on the documentation of the proximate nutrient composition, impact on the animal feed industry, consumer acceptance, and safety of insect meal as animal feed.

2. Chemical composition of different insect meals

Insects at all stages of their lives are potentially rich in protein [8]. Frantic efforts by researchers have dealt with different insect species, as indicated in **Table 1**. The protein content of insect meals varies considerably, from around 39% up to 64.4% even when the meals are based on the same insect species. The nutrient concentration of insects depends on their life stage as well as the rearing conditions and the composition of the growth media used for insect production [3, 20].

Insect spp.	DM	CP	EE	Ash	CF	Citation
Tenebrio molitor L.	94.56	52.18	32.19			[10]
Gryllus assimilis	90.15	58.14	29.52			[10]
T. molitor	99.20	58.80	17.1			[11]
Hermetia illucens	98.9	58.4	11.6			[11]
Periplaneta americana	94.6	64.4	23.6	3.98	4.36	[12]
Hydrous cavistanum	86.3	41.9	38.3	1.88	14.7	[12]
Zophobas morio	96.8	42.0	41.7	5.53	6.28	[12]
Locusta migratoria	91.9	58.5	12.7	4.56	12.7	[12]
Gryllus testaceus	92.2	53.3	22.6	5.05	8.98	[12]
Musca domesticus	93.8	54.8	21.7	6.78	9.65	[12]
Brachytrupes spp.		62.6	12.2	4.9	13.3	[13]
G. assimilis		56.0	32.0		7.6	[14]
Ruspolia nitidula		40.8	46.3	3.3	5.9	[15]
Macrotermes nigeriensis		37.5	48.0	3.2	5.0	[16]
Allomyrina dichotoma		54.2	20.20	3.9	4.0	[17]
H. illucens		39.0	32.6	14.6	12.4	[18]
Musa domestica	96.77	40.12	6.88	15.88	10.97	[19]

Table 1.
Summarized major chemical composition of different insect meals.

3. Impact of insect meal in the animal feed industry

In general, insects can be utilized for human and animal feed because of their high nutritive value [21]. Several studies have indicated that insect meal can be utilized to substitute soybean and fish meal in animal diets [22–26]. This is because these are rich sources of macro and micronutrients [27]. For instance, the black soldier fly (BSF) *Hermetia illucens* larvae has a protein content of 37–63 g/100 g and fat levels of 20–40 g/100 g with balanced fatty acids and amino acids profiles [9, 28]. Furthermore, grasshoppers (*Ruspolia nitidula* Linnaeus) family *Tettigoniidae* contains 36–40 g/100 g crude protein, 41–43 g/100 g fat, 10–13 g/100 g dietary fiber, and 2.6–3.9 g/100 g ash on a dry matter basis [29]. In addition, insects are excellent sources of minerals like potassium, calcium, iron, phosphorous, zinc, and magnesium and also vitamins covering riboflavin, thiamine, niacin, and vitamin B12 [30–32].

Furthermore, Onsongo et al. [24] reported that broiler chickens and quails fed on BSF larvae meal had a satisfactory taste, aroma, and nutritional composition of the meat. This denotes that BSF larval meal can be suitable to be incorporated in poultry diets. Also, insects have been fed to fish yielding good growth performance and feed conversion [33]. In addition, piglets fed with BSF larval meal exhibited good results on growth performance, with insignificant effects on blood

Pig age	Insect species	Feed inclusion levels	Results	Citation
Weaned pigs	*Tenebrio molitor*	0, 1.5, 3.0, 4.5, and 6.0% replacement of soybean meal	Linear increase in BW, ADG, ADFI, DM, and CP digestibility	[44]
Weaned female pigs	*Hermetia illucens*	0, 30, and 60% replacement of soybean meal	Linear increase in ADFI no effect on growth	[26]
Barrows	*H. illucens*	50, 75, and 100% replacement of soybean meal	No effect on base meat quality measures, increased juiciness ($P < 0.05$); higher back fat PUFA contents ($P < 0.05$)	[45]
Weaned pigs	*T. molitor*	0, 5, and 10% replacement of soybean	AID of all AAs, except aspartic acid, was lower at 10% inclusion than at the control diet	[46]
Growing pig	Dried BSF larvae meal	0, 9, 12, 14.5, and 18.5% replacing fish meal	Growth performance was not affected	[47]
Finishing pigs	Dried *H. illucens* larvae powder	0, 4, and 8% replacing soybean meal	BW and BWG at 4% inclusion was higher and FCR was lower than at 0 and 8% inclusion	[48]
Weaned piglets	*H. illucens* larvae oil	0, 2, 4, and 6% replacing corn oil	Evaluated biochemical parameters were not affected, except cholesterol that increased linearly at higher inclusion levels. Hematological parameters were not affected, but platelet count tended to linearly increase at higher inclusion levels	[49]
Nursing piglets	*H. illucens* larva	0 and 3.5% replacing fishmeal	Evaluated hematological and biochemical parameters were not affected	[50]
Growing quails	Defatted *H. illucens* meal		Reported no difference in average daily feed intake	[51]
Broiler chickens	Mopane worn (*Imbrasia belina meal*)	0, 4, 8, and 12% replacing soybean oil	Dietary inclusion levels of *I. belina* meal up to 12% had a positive effect on growth performance, meat quality, and sensory attributes	[52]
Broiler chickens	*Musca domestica*	0, 75, 50, and 25% replacing fish meal	No significant effect ($P > 0.05$) to the feed intake	[19]
Quails	*H. illucens*	0, 10, and 15% substituting soybean oil	No significant difference in daily gains to control	[52]
Broiler chickens	*T. molitor*	0, 50, 100, and 150%	Live weight and feed intake of broiler chickens improved with increasing levels of *T. molitor*	[53]
Broiler chickens	*H. illucens* and *Arthrospira platensis*	50%	Increased live weight of broiler chickens	[54]

Pig age	Insect species	Feed inclusion levels	Results	Citation
Broilers chickens	*H. illucens*	0, 5, 10, and 15%	Live weight showed linear and quadratic responses to increasing levels of *H. illucens*	[55]
Muscovy duck	*H. Illucens*	0, 3, 6, and 9%	Live weight and average daily gain showed quadratic response to increasing *H. illucens*	[56]

DM, dry matter; CP, crude protein; BW, body weight; BWG, body weight gain; FCR, food conversion ratio; ADG, average daily gain; ADFI, average daily feed intake; AA, amino acids; AIA, apparent ileal digestibility; PUFA, polyunsaturated fatty acid.

Table 2.
Summary of effect of insect diet on growth performance of different animal species.

profiles [26]. However, generally, the use of BSF larval meal has been proven to be an excellent constituent of animal feed [23–26].

High nutritional value, minimal space requirements, and low environmental impact combine to make insects an appealing option for animal feed [34]. Another major advantage is that insects are already used for the natural part of many animal diets [35]. Insect-based animal feeds are particularly attractive when considering the cost of standard feeds, currently accounting for 70% of livestock-production expenses [36].

The most promising, well-studied candidates for industrial feed production are black soldier flies, larvae, yellow mealworms, silkworms, grasshoppers, and termites [37]. Such previous research has revealed that insect meal can partially replace commercial soybean or fish meal in broiler feed, particularly as protein sources. In addition, Pretorius [38] reported that broiler chicken fed with housefly larvae increased their average daily gain, carcass weight, and total feed intake. More so, a recent study by [9] asserted that broilers fed on BSF meal improved their growth performance. With regards to nutritional value, insect diets improved meat products' taste. Also, Marono et al. [39] reported that laying hens fed on insect larvae meal exhibited no negative effect on feed intake, feed conversion efficiency, immune status, egg production, and health. Smallholder farmers in Asia and Africa frequently utilize insect diets on fish production [37]. Mealworms and housefly-larvae meal can substitute up to 40–80% and 75% of fishmeal in Nile tilapia/standard catfish (*Ameiurus melas* Raf.) diets without any detrimental effects, respectively [40, 41]. Replacing a fish meal with black-soldier-fly larvae meal in diets does not alter the odor, flavor, or texture of Atlantic salmon (*Salmo salar*) [42]. Another viable alternative to a fish meal is silkworm pupa, which was tested successfully for African catfish (*Clarias gariepinus*) fingerling diets [43]. More so, some other outcomes on insects to benefit the industry are presented in **Table 2**.

4. Consumer's acceptance of insect-based animal feeds

The utilization of insect meal to replace unaffordable fish, animal, or plant protein ingredients in feeds is socially acceptable. This is because, naturally, fish and poultry are usually seen feeding on insects, for example, in the case of our free-range poultry production systems [53, 57], which roam around in search of feed. More so, various insects have higher protein levels than conventional fish and soybean meals [58] and are comparable in performance with conventional protein sources when completely or partially replaced with fish protein in poultry diets [59]. With the fact that protein is the most costly ingredient in livestock diets, the use of insects sounds like a positive novel idea [60, 61].

The consumer's acceptance of meat products derived from animals-fed insects ought to be put into account. Before introducing insects as a new ingredient, it is necessary to establish the current perceptions of the targeted processors, traders, and poultry farmers. This is because farmers' perceptions of technology characteristics significantly affect their adoption decisions [62]. A few studies surveyed the consumer's readiness to buy animal products that originated from animals fed with insect meal [63, 64].

5. Chitin content

Chitin is a polysaccharide (linear polymer of β-(1–4)*N*-acetyl-glucosamine units) of the exoskeleton of arthropods [65]. However, chitin negatively affects the digestibility and nutritional traits of insects. In addition, it has been considered as indigestible fiber for the time in memorial. Chitin is the utmost form of fiber in insects [66], however, the nitrogen absence is also analyzed by the Kjeldahl method as a crude protein. It is, however, included in the nitrogen-to-protein conversion factor of 6.25, which overvalued protein content. For this reason, Janssen et al. [67] suggested a conversion factor of 5.60 ± 0.39. However, in some birds like chickens, the gastrointestinal tract (GIT) excretes the enzyme chitinase [68] which degrades chitin into its derivatives chitosan, chitooligosaccharides, and chitooligomers that are assimilated with easy into bloodstreams [68, 69]. Average chitin yields were 18.01 and 4.92% of dry weight from the exuvium and whole body of the *Tenebrio molitor* larvae [70]. The chitin composition depends on species and development stadium of the insect [66].

However, chitin has a positive effect on the operation of the immune system of poultry, which could reduce the use of antibiotics [1]. The prebiotic effect of chitin was observed by [71, 72] in increasing caecal production of butyric acid and [73] in improving the immune response of birds or due to reduction of albumin to globulin ratio [74]. In addition, chitin and its derivatives can aid to sustain a balanced and healthy GIT microbiota that keeps the amounts of potentially pathogenic bacteria (e.g., *Escherichia coli* and *Salmonella typhimurium*) low [75] and decreases the risk of intestinal diseases. By reducing the number of pathogenic microbiota, chitin encourages the proliferation of commensal bacteria. A positive effect of chitin was reported by [36] who also stated that a diet containing 3% of chitin decreased *E. coli* and *Salmonella* spp. in the 380 intestines. Chitin also has antifungal and antimicrobial properties [76].

6. Nutrient digestibility

Evaluating digestibility is a means to come up with an approximation of nutrient availability in a feed. In this regards, Woods et al. [77] reported that *H. illucens* larvae fed to quails have higher apparent digestibility for dry matter and organic matter to the control fed group. However, Bovera et al. [78] showed that the ileal digestibility coefficient of dry matter and organic matter in broiler fed *T. molitor* was lower by 2% than fed soybean diet. In addition, Cutrignelli et al. [79] reported reduced coefficients of the apparent ileal digestibility (AID) of dry and organic matter on laying hens fed *H. illucens* meal diet. These reductions were due to the strong decrease of the crude protein digestibility linked to the availability of chitin in the insect meals, which deleteriously influences the crude protein digestibility. However, no difference was observed between digestibility coefficients of the dry matter of *T. molitor* meal and *H. illucens* meal [80]. More so, Woods et al. [77]

observed a higher apparent metabolizable energy for *H. illucens* larvae fed quail compared well to the control fed group. On similar results [81] did not find the differences among *T. molitor* oil and palm oil on AID of crude fat, and metabolizable energy. Furthermore, the apparent metabolizable energy of the *T. molitor* meal and *H. illucens* meal [80] was higher than all the ingredients mainly utilized in the poultry diet [39], substituted 500 g kg^{-1} of a maize meal-based diet with *M. domestica* larvae meal for 3-week old broiler chickens and detected a crude protein digestibility coefficient of 0.69. However, De-Marco et al. [80] detected no difference in the digestibility coefficient of the crude protein between *T. molitor* and *H. illucens*. In their study, Schiavone et al. [82] observed that there was no effect on apparent crude protein digestibility in chickens fed *T. molitor* oil as a total replacement for palm oil. Whilst, Bovera et al. [78] and Schiavone et al. [82] reported 8.2% and lower crude protein digestibility on chickens fed *T. molitor* larvae respectively, compared to soybean diet. De-Marco et al. [80], found that the (AID) of amino acids in the *T. molitor* meal was higher and showed less variation than in the *H. illucens* meal. According to the afore-mentioned results, insect meals can be an alternative crude protein source for soybean meals or fishmeal.

7. Safety in utilization of insect meals

Utilization of insects as constituents in livestock feed should consider safe due to the fact that they contain toxic substances secreted by the exocrine gland [83]. Just as in plants and animal feed, some insects are not safe to eat, they trigger allergic reactions. For instance, African silkworm (*Anaphe venata*) pupae have a thiaminase which causes thiamine deficiency [84]. In addition, *T. molitor* contains toxic benzoquinone compounds secreted by the defensive gland [85]. This benzoquinone is toxic to humans and animals, hence affecting cellular respiration resulting in kidney destruction, and has a carcinogenic effect [85]. However, insects may have antibiotic resistance genes [86] indicating that they can be filled with disease-causing organisms or mycotoxin from adulterated diets. More so, Wynants et al. [87] affirmed the contamination of wheat bran by the *Salmonella* spp. in *T. molitor* larvae. However, it is imperative to consistently monitor microbial pathogens of the substrate and the larvae in order to reduce pathogens in the *T. molitor*. Interestingly, Van Broekhoven et al. [88] reported that *T. molitor* larvae fed with diets contaminated with the mycotoxin deoxynivalenol were not affected in their growth and degraded the mycotoxin.

Besides, mycotoxins, insect feed can be contaminated with heavy metals, pesticides [89]. Mycotoxins from feed or substrate for insects rearing can negatively affect the growth, inhibit larval development or increase mortality of insects. More so, consumption of mycotoxin-contaminated insects can present a risk to animals. However, Schrogel et al. [90], reported no accumulation of mycotoxin in experiments fed with various insect species. Furthermore, Charlton et al. [91] reported that heavy metals accumulate in resultant insects. However, of the 1140 compounds measured, only seven were detected in the larvae, with Cd posing the greatest risk [91]. The *T. molitor* and *H. illucens* larvae consume feeds containing mycotoxins and pesticides, the removal of these would render the resultant larvae free from toxins [92, 93]. More so, Purschke et al. [94] affirmed that there was no build-up of pesticides in BSF larvae raised on substrates spiked with pesticides. As a result, this renders it safe to be used in animal feed diets.

Some insects contain repellent or toxic chemicals, which they use as their defense mechanism. Grasshoppers spit brown juice as a means of defense while laybugs protect themselves from predators by releasing toxic fluid hemolymph.

This yellowish fluid released from the leg joints is toxic in nature. Some insects are reported to transmit zoonotic agents such as bacteria, viruses, parasites, and fungi as vectors. According to [95] cases of botulism, parasites and food poisoning have been reported in using insect meal. In management, these health risks, proper processing, handling, and storage are a necessity in order to prevent contamination and spoilage. However, it is imperative to apply decontamination methods and shelf-life stability of insect meals in order to ensure and achieve marketability and food and feed safety.

8. Production and availability of insect meal

Insects have some valuable biological traits, which include being prolific, high feed conversion rate, and easy to raise with low feed cost [96]. According to [51] insects need less amount of feed for the production of 1 kg biomass, have higher fecundity, for instance, the common house cricket lays up to 1500 eggs over a period of about a month. Insect species are efficient feed converters as they are cold-blooded [51] and do not use energy to maintain body temperature [53]. Insects effectively utilize water and, in most cases, the feed is the main source of water [97]. Generally, the breeding of insects does not require complex infrastructure and their care is simple [98]. Insects propagation can be on several substrates, for example, cereals, decomposing organic materials, fruit or vegetables, poultry, pigs and cattle manure, industry by-products, or waste products, which would be environmental problems [51, 99]. According to [100, 101] utilization of insect meals or larvae meals can reduce the cost of poultry feed when nurtured on bio-waste. Insects can convert waste into valuable biomass [102] and convert low-quality plant waste into high-quality crude protein, fat, and energy in a short time [3]. Insects can effectively convert low-grade organic waste into high-quality protein. They utilize the organic waste, which could otherwise end up on dumpsites, causing environmental pollution. Insects have higher feed conversion efficiency. Most insects are produced on organic wastes or material that could not be consumed by humans. In their production, insects use minimal space, in the rearing process. Reports indicate that insects contribute less greenhouse gases than pigs and cattle [37].

The other benefit is the larvae's ability to decrease bacterial growth in the manure and thus reduce odor [97] *H. illucens* larvae has a 66% potential waste reduction and also waste reduction of 51–80% was recorded on pig, chicken, and kitchen waste [103]. Insect farming can also provide environmental benefits. Feeding waste materials to insects protects air, land, and water from potential contamination [104]. For example, the black soldier fly (*H. illucens* L.) (Diptera: Stratiomyidae), can be fed food waste that would typically be placed in landfills [105]. Accordingly, digestion of these materials suppresses noxious odors [105] greenhouse gases [106], and pathogens [107]. Furthermore, less land, water, and space are needed to produce insects, such as the black soldier fly, than traditional animal production [107]. Other benefits include fast development time (e.g., black soldier fly can develop to harvestable size within 14 days) [108], versus beef (e.g., 12–18 months of feeding to reach the needed weight to slaughter) [109]. It is also worth noting that the full insect is edible unlike beef (48.5%) [36]. Because of the ability of the black soldier fly to consume a variety of organic wastes, while offering benefits to the environment, it is now viewed as the "crown jewel" of the insect.

Insects' growth rate depends on microclimate. The optimal temperature for most insect species rearing is 27–30°C [110]. The insect's larvae are the most effective for production and it is possible to produce more than 180 kg of live weight of *H. illucens* larvae in 42 days from 1 m^2 [110]. The insect market for animal feed is continually increasing globally, especially focused on *T. molitor* larvae (mealworm).

T. molitor and *H. illucens* (black soldier fly) are two of the most promising insect species for commercial exploitation and for use in poultry feeds [110] their production is seamless and well understood [111].

Even though raising insects seem to be a positive move, there is a dearth of information with regards to insect production methods and technologies, mainly in mass production [112–114]. This may be due to the fact that private companies hardly share that kind of information as they are in business. However, indigenous technical knowledge is mainly utilized in raising these insects, eventually becoming the basis of any technological improvement. For instance, in Indonesia, a complete guide on how *H. illucens* on medium-scale production has been circulated [115]. General, insect husbandry includes two main distinct units, which include the maintenance of the breeding colonies and the growing larvae [28]. In the event that business deals with adult insects, this requires more space for rearing purposes. As this implies to where crickets are raised [116]. Improved systems usually include an area to process insects and improve resultant products. Production wastes, like substrate remains and frass, may be utilized to come up with fertilizers in a devoted facility, hence leading to circularity and sustainability.

Insects can thrive in thickly populated areas, which permits mass production even in limited spaces. Generally, larvae and pupae are retained together with a nourishing substrate in small trays made of diverse materials like wood, high-density polyethylene, or fiberglass. According to [116] trays for fattening *T. molitor* larvae are standard ones measuring $65 \times 50 \times 15$ cm^3 box, which are handled with ease and are deep enough to avert larvae or adults from fleeing. A recent study by Thevenot et al. [114] reported that a mill was designed to produce 17 tones of *T. molitor* annually with a density of 5 larvae cm^{-2}.

Currently, insect raising is appealingly increasing awareness in developed countries, which are not enthusiastically normally involved in harvesting insects. This involves countries like Europe and the United States of America. As a result, promoting insect-based products to increase their market share. Indeed, insect husbandry linked with economic benefits produce food and feed ingredients that can benefit the developing and developed nations [117].

9. Conclusion

Insects pose an attractive opportunity to come up with novel sustainable protein source in monogastric animal diets taking into account their nutritive value, biosafety, and consumer acceptance. In addition, they also represent a means of converting food waste biomasses/streams into valued feed materials. However, it appears that there is nothing much barring us from utilizing insect meals as feed material. As a result, we need to get started and reduce the feed costs and also get rid of other insect limitations in their use as animal feed. Insect farming has great potential with regards to sustainably providing feed for the livestock. It can be concluded that insects can be an excellent alternative to partly replace soybean and fishmeal. However, further technological development of this sector and monitoring of the effects of these developments are needed. Also, further exploration is needed to assess the estimation equations parameters tied to these insect species.

Acknowledgements

The authors would like to extend their gratitude to Gwanda State University for granting us an opportunity, resources, facilities to work on this chapter.

Our appreciation also goes to the Animal Feed Science and Nutrition-Health Environment for affording us the opportunity to make this contribution. This research did not receive any external funding from outside.

Conflict of interest

The authors declare no potential conflict of interest.

Thanks

Our appreciation also goes to the Animal Feed Science and Nutrition-Health Environment for affording us the opportunity to make this contribution.

Author details

Sipho Moyo* and Busani Moyo
Faculty of Life Science, Department of Animal Science, Gwanda State University, Filabusi Epoch Mine, Zimbabwe

*Address all correspondence to: sipho.moyo@gsu.ac.zw

References

[1] Food Agriculture Organization (FAO). Insects as Animal Feed. Available from: http://www.fao.org/3/i3253e/i3253e07.pdf [Accessed: 2 November 2021]

[2] Van Huis A, Oonincx DGAB. The environmental sustainability of insect as food and feed. A review. Agronomy for Sustainable Development. 2017;**37**:43. DOI: 10.1007/s/3593-017-0452-8

[3] Makkar HP, Tran G, Heuzé V, Ankers P. State-of-the-art on use of insects as animal feed. Animal Feed Science and Technology. 2014;**197**:1-33

[4] Gasco L, Finke M, van Huis A. Can diets containing insects promote animal health? Journal of Insects as Food and Feed. 2018;**4**:5

[5] Khan SH. Recent advances in the role of insects as an alternative protein source in poultry nutrition. Journal of Applied Animal Research. 2018; **46**:1144-1157

[6] Belforti M, Gai F, Lussiana C, Renna M, Malfatto V, Rotolo L. *Tenebrio molitor* meal in rainbow trout (*Oncorhynchus mykiss*) diets: Effects on animal performance, nutrient digestibility and chemical composition of fillets. Italian Journal of Animal Science. 2015;**14**:670-675

[7] Renna M, Schiavone A, Gai F, Dabbou S, Lussiana C, Malfatto V. Evaluation of the suitability of a partially defatted black soldier fly (*Hermetia illucens* L.) larvae meal as an ingredient for rainbow trout (*Oncorhynchus mykiss* Walbaum) diets. Journal of Animal Science and Biotechnology. 2017;**8**:957-969

[8] Bovera F, Piccolo G, Gasco L, Marono S, Loponte R, Vassalotti G, et al. Yellow meal larvae (*Tenebrio molitor*) as a possible alternative to soybean meal in broiler diets. British Poultry Science. 2015;**56**(5):569-575. DOI: 10.1080/00071668.2015.1080815

[9] Schiavone A, De Marco M, Martínez S, Dabbou S, Renna M, Madrid J. Nutritional value of a partially defatted and a highly defatted black soldier fly larvae (*Hermetia illucens* L.) meal for broiler chickens: Apparent nutrient digestibility, apparent metabolizable energy and apparent ileal amino acid digestibility. Journal of Animal Science and Biotechnology. 2017;**8**:897-905

[10] Dourado LRB, Lopes PM, Silva VK, Carvalho FLA, Maura FAS, Silva LB, et al. Chemical composition and nutrient digestibility of insect meal for broilers. Annals of the Brazilian Academy of Sciences. 2020;**90**:3. DOI: 10.1590/0001-37652020200764

[11] Marono S, Piccolo G, Loponte R, Meo CD, Attia YA, Nozza A, et al. In vitro crude protein digestibility of *Tenebrio molitor* and *Hermetia illucens* insect meals and its correlation with chemical compostion traits. Italian Journal of Animal Science. 2015; **14**:3889. DOI: 10.408I/ijas.2015.3889

[12] Kovitvadhi A, Chundang P, Thongprajukaew K, Tirawattanawainich C, Srikachar S, Chotimanothum B. Potential of insect meals as protein sources for meat-type ducks based on in vitro digestibility. Animals. 2019;**9**:155. DOI: 10.3390/ani9040155

[13] Akullo J, Agea JG, Obaa BB, Okwee-Acai J, Nokimbugwe D. Nutritional composition of commonly consumed edible insects in the Lango sub-region of northern Uganda. International Food Research Journal. 2018;**25**:159-166

[14] Adamkova A, Ml'cek J, Kou'rimska L, Borkovcova M, Busina T, Adamek M, et al. Nutritional potential of selected insect species reared on the Island of Sumatra. International Journal of Environmental Research and Public Health. 2017;**14**:521

[15] Bbosa T, Ndagire CT, Mukisa IM, Fiaboe KKM, Nakimbugwe D. Nutritional characteristics of selected insects in Uganda for use as alternative protein sources in food and feed. Journal of Insect Science. 2019;**19**:23

[16] Omotoso OT. Nutrition composition, mineral analysis and antinutrient factors of *Oryctes rhinoceros* L. (Scarabaeidae: Coleoptea) and winged termites, *Macrotermes nigeriensis Sjostedt* (Termitidae: Isoptera). Brazilian Journal of Applied Science and Technology. 2015;**8**:97-106

[17] Ghosh S, Lee SM, Jung C, Meyer-Rochow VB. Nutritional composition of five commercial edible insects in South Korea. Journal of Asia-Pacific Entomology. 2017; **20**:686-694

[18] Nyakeri EM, Ogola HJ, Ayieko MA, Amimo FA. An open system for farming black soldier fly larvae as a source of proteins for small scale poultry and fish production. Journal of Insects as Food and Feed. 2017;**3**:51-56

[19] Dillak SYFG, Suryatni NPF, Handayani HT, Temu ST, Nastiti HP, Osa DB, et al. The effect of fed maggot meal as a supplement of finisher broiler chickens. Earth and Environmental Science. 2019;**260**:2-6

[20] Oonincx DGAB, Van Broekhoven S, Van Huis A, Van Loon JJA. Feed conversion, survival and development, and composition of four insect species on diets composed of food by-products. PLoS One. 2015;**10**(12):e0144601

[21] Klunder HC, Wolkers-Rooijackers J, Kopela JM, Noute MJR. Microbial aspects of processing and storage of edible insects. Food Control. 2012;**26**:628-631. DOI: 10.1016/j.foodcont.2012.02.013

[22] Tran G, Heuze V, Makkar HPS. Insects in fish diets. Animal Frontiers. 2015;**5**:37-44

[23] Iaconisi V, Marono S, Parisi G, Gasco L, Genovese L, Maricchiolo G, et al. Dietary inclusion of *Tenebrio molitor* larvae meal: effects on growth performance and final quality traits of blackspot sea bream (*Pagellus bogaraveo*). Aquaculture. 2017;**476**:49-58. DOI: 10.1016/j.aquaculture.2017.04.007

[24] Onsongo VO, Osuga IM, Gachuiri CK, Wachira AM, Miano DM, Tanga CM, et al. Insects for income generation through animal feed: Effect of dietary replacement of soybean and fish meal with black soldier fly meal on broiler growth and economic performance. Journal of Economic Entomology. 2018;**111**:1966-1973. DOI: 10.1093/jee/toy118

[25] Van der Fels-Klerx HJ, Camenzuli L, Belluco S, Meijer N, Ricci A. Food safety issues related to uses of insects for feeds and foods. Comprehensive Reviews in Food Science and Food Safety. 2018;**17**:1172-1183. DOI: 10.1111/1541-4337.12385

[26] Biasato I, Renna M, Gai F, Dabbou S, Meneguz M, Perona G, et al. Partially defatted black soldier fly larva meal inclusion in piglet diets: Effects on the growth performance, nutrient digestibility, blood profile, gut morphology and histological features. Journal of Animal Science and Biotechnology. 2019;**10**:2-6. DOI: 10.1186/s40104-019-0325-x.13

[27] Finke M, Oonincx DGAB. Nutrient content of insects. In: Van Huis A, Tomberlin JK, editors. Insects as Food and Feed: From Production to

Consumption. Netherlands: Wageningen Academic Publishers; 2017. pp. 290-316

[28] Halloran A, Flore R, Vantomme P, Roos N. Insects and human nutrition. In: Halloran A, Flore R, Vantomme P, Roos N, editors. Edible Insects in Sustainable Food Systems. Cham: Springer; 2018. pp. 83-92. DOI: 10.1007/978-3-319-74011-9

[29] Ssepuuya G, Mukisa IM, Nakimbugwe D. Nutritional composition, quality and shelf life stability of processed *Ruspolia nitidula* (edible grass hoppers). Food Science & Nutrition. 2016;**5**:103-112. DOI: 10.1002/fsn3.369

[30] Kourimska L, Adamkova A. Nutritional and sensory quality of edible insects. Nutrition and Food Science Journal. 2016;**4**:22-26

[31] Spranghers T, Ottoboni M, Klootwijk C, Ovyn A, Deboosere S, De Meulenaer B, et al. Nutritional composition of black soldier fly (*Hermetia illucens*) prepupae reared on different organic waste substrates. Journal of the Science of Food and Agriculture. 2017;**97**:2594-2600. DOI: 10.1002/jsfa.8081

[32] Akhtar Y, Isman MB. Insects as an alternative protein source. In: Rickey YY, editor. Proteins in Food Processing. Canada: Woodhead Publishing Series in Food Science, Technology and Nutrition; 2018. pp. 263-288

[33] Devic E, Leschen W, Murray F, Little DC. Growth performance, feed utilization and body composition of advanced nursing Nile tilapia (*Oreochromis niloticus*) fed diets containing Black Soldier Fly (*Hermetia illucens*) larvae meal. Aquaculture Nutrition. 2018;**24**:416-423

[34] Kim TK, Yang HI, Kim YB, Kim HW, Choi YS. Edible insects as a protein source: A review of public perception, processing, technology, and research trends. Food Science of Animal Resources. 2019;**39**(4):521-540. DOI: 10.5851/kosfa.2019.e53

[35] Veldkamp T, Bosch G. Insects: A protein-rich feed ingredient in pig and poultry diets. Animal Frontiers. 2015;**5**:45-50

[36] van Huis A, van Itterbeeck J, Klunder H, Mertens E, Halloran A, Muir G, et al. Edible Insects: Future Prospects for Food and Feed Security. Rome: Food and Agriculture Organization of the United Nations; 2013

[37] Dobermann D, Swift JA, Field LM. Opportunities and hurdles of edible insects for food and feed. Nutrition Bulletin. 2017;**42**:293-308

[38] Pretorius Q. The evaluation of larvae of *Musca domestica* (common house fly) as protein source for broiler production [Ph.D. dissertation]. Stellenbosch, Republic of South Africa: Stellenbosch University; 2011

[39] Marono S, Loponte R, Lombardi P, Vassalotti G, Pero ME, Russo F, et al. Productive performance and blood profiles of laying hens fed *Hermetia illucens* larvae meal as total replacement of soybean meal from 24 to 45 weeks of age. Poultry Science. 2017;**96**:1783-1790

[40] Roncarati A, Gasco L, Parisi G, Terova G. Growth performance of common catfish (*Ameiurus melas* Raf.) fingerlings fed mealworm (*Tenebrio molitor*) diet. Journal of Insects as Food and Feed. 2015;**1**:233-240

[41] Wang L, Li J, Jin JN, Zhu F, Roffeis M, Zhang XZ. A comprehensive evaluation of replacing fishmeal with housefly (*Musca domestica*) maggot meal in the diet of Nile tilapia (*Oreochromis niloticus*): Growth performance, flesh quality, innate immunity and water environment. Aquatic Nutrition. 2017;**23**:983-993

[42] Lock ER, Arsiwalla T, Waagbo R. Insect larvae meal as an alternative source of nutrients in the diet of Atlantic salmon (*Salmo salar*) posts molt. Aquatic Nutrition. 2016; **22**:1202-1213

[43] Kurbanov AR, Milusheva RY, Rashidova SS, Kamilov BG. Effect of replacement of fish meal with silkworm (*Bombyx mori*) pupa protein on the growth of *Clarias gariepinus* Fingerling. International Journal of Fisheries and Aquatic Studies. 2015;**2**:25-27

[44] Jin XH, Heo PS, Hong JS, Kim NJ, Kim YY. Supplementation of dried mealworm (*Tenebrio molitor* larva) on growth performance, nutrient digestibility and blood profiles in weaning pigs. Asian-Australasian Journal of Animal Sciences. 2016; **29**:979-986

[45] Altmann BA, Neumann C, Rothstein S, Liebert F, Mörlein D. Do dietary soy alternatives lead to pork quality improvements or drawbacks? A look into micro-alga and insect protein in swine diets. Meat Science. 2019;**153**:26-34

[46] Meyer S, Gessner DK, Braune MS, Friedhoff T, Most E, Horing M, et al. Comprehensive evaluation of the metabolic effects of insect meal from *Tenebrio molitor* L. in growing pigs by transcriptomics, metabolomics and lipidomics. Journal of Animal Science and Biotechnology. 2020;**11**:20

[47] Chia SY, Tanga CM, Osuga IM, Alaru AO, Mwangi DM, Githinji M, et al. Effect of dietary replacement of fishmeal by insect meal on growth performance, blood profiles and economics of growing pigs in Kenya. Animals. 2019;**9**:19

[48] Yu M, Li ZM, Chen WD, Rong T, Wang G, Li JH, et al. Use of *Hermetia illucens* larvae as a dietary protein source: Effects on growth performance, carcass traits, and meat quality in finishing pigs. Meat Science. 2019;**158**:2-6

[49] Van Heugten E, Martinez G, McComb A, Koutsos E. Black soldier fly (*Hermetia illucens*) larvae oil improves growth performance of nursery pigs. Journal of Animal Science. 2019;**97**:1

[50] Driemeyer H. Evaluation of black soldier fly (*Hermetia illucens*) larvae as an alternative protein source in pig creep diets in relation to production, blood and manure microbiology parameters [MSc thesis]. Stellenbosch, South Africa: Stellenbosch University; 2016. p. 99

[51] Cullere M, Tasoniero G, Giaccone V, Miotti-Scapin R, Claey E, Dr Smet S, et al. Black soldier fly as dietary protein source for broiler quails: Apparent digestibility, excretal microbial load, feed choice, performance, carcass and meat traits. Animal. 2016;**10**(12): 1923-1930

[52] Moyo S, Masika PJ, Muchenje V, Jaja IF. Effect of *Imbrasia belina* meal on growth performance, quality characteristics and sensory attributes of broiler chicken meal. Italian Journal of Animal Science. 2020;**19**(1):1450-1461

[53] Biasato I, Gasco L, De Marco M, Renna M, Rotolo L, Dabbou S, et al. Yellow mealworm larvae (*Tenebrio molitor*) inclusion in diets for male broiler chickens: Effects on growth performance, gut morphology and histological findings. Poultry Science. 2018;**97**:540-548

[54] Altmann BA, Neumann C, Velten S, Liebert F, Mörlein D. Meat quality derived from high inclusion of a micro-alga or insect meal as an alternative protein source in poultry diets: A pilot study. Foods (Basel, Switzerland). 2018;**7**:34

[55] Dabbou S, Gai F, Biasato I, Gasco L, Schiavone A. Black soldier fly defatted

meal as dietary protein source of broiler chickens: Effect on growth performance, blood traits, gut morphology and histology features. Journal of Animal Science and Biotechnology. 2018;**9**:48. DOI: 10.1186/s40104-018-0266-9

[56] Gariglio M, Dabbou S, Biasato I, Capucchio MT, Colombino E, Hernandez F, et al. Nutritional effect of the dietary inclusion of partially defatted *Hermetia illucens* larva meal in Muscovy duck. Journal of Animal Biotechnology. 2019;**10**:10-37. DOI: 10.1186/s40104-019-6344-7

[57] Sebatta C, Ssepuuya G, Sikahwa E, Mugisha J, Diiro G, Sengendo M, et al. Farmers' acceptance of insects as an alternative protein source in poultry feeds. International Journal of Agricultural Research, Innovation and Technology. 2018;**8**(2):32-41. DOI: 10.3329/ijarit.v8i2.40553

[58] Anand H, Ganguly A, Haldar P. Potential value of acridids as high protein supplement for poultry feed. International Journal of Poultry Science. 2008;**7**(7):722-725

[59] Moreki J, Tiroesele B, Chiripasi S. Prospects of utilizing insects as alternative sources of protein in poultry diets in Botswana: A review. Journal of Animal Science Advances. 2012;**2**(8): 649-658

[60] Maurer V, Holinger M, Amsler Z, Früh B, Wohlfahrt J, Stamer A, et al. Replacement of soybean cake by *Hermetia illucens* meal in diets for layers. Journal of Insects as Food and Feed. 2016;**2**(2):83-90

[61] Niassy S, Ekesi S. Contribution to the knowledge of entomophagy in Africa. Journal of Insects as Food and Feed. 2016;**2**(3):137-138

[62] Mbaka JN, Mwangi M, Mwangi MN. Banana farming as a business: The role of tissue cultured planting materials in Kenya. Journal of Applied Biosciences. 2008;**9**(1):354-361

[63] Verbeke W, Spranghers T, De Clercq P, De Smet S, Sas B, Eeckhout M. Insect in animal feed: acceptance and determinants among farmers, agriculture sector, stakeholders and Citizens. Animal Feed Science and Technology. 2015;**204**:72-87

[64] Szendo K, Naggy MZ, Toth K. Consumer acceptance of meat from animals reared on insect meal feed. Animals. 2020;**10**:1213. DOI: 10/3390/ani10081312

[65] Sanchez-Muros MJ, Barroso FG, Manzano-Agugliaro F. Insect meal a renewable source of food for animal feeding: A review. Journal of Cleaner Production. 2014;**65**:16-27

[66] Al-Qazzaz MFA, Ismail D, Akit H, Idris LH. Effect of using insect larvae meal as a complete protein source on quality and productivity characteristics of laying hens. Revista Brasileira de Zootecnia. 2016;**45**(9):518-523

[67] Janssen RH, Vinken JP, van Den Broek LAM, Fogliano V, Lakemond CMM. Nitrogen-to-protein conversion factors for three edible insects; *Tenebrio molitor*, *Alphitobius diaperinus* and *Hermetia illucens*. Journal of Agricultural and Food Chemistry. 2010;**65**(11):2275-2278. DOI: 10.1021/acs.jafc.7600471

[68] Tabata E, Kashimura A, Wakita S, Ohno M, Sakaguchi M, Sugahara Y, et al. Gastric and intestinal protease resistance of chicken acidic chitinase nominates chitin-containing organisms for alternative whole edible diets for poultry. Scientific Reports. 2017;**7**:6662. DOI: 10.1038/541598-017-07146-3

[69] Borrelli L, Coretti L, Dipineto L, Bovera F, Monna F, Chiariotti L, et al. Insect-based diet, a promising

nutritional source, modulates gut microbiota composition and short chain fatty acids (SCFAS) production in laying hens. Scientific Reports. 2017;7:16269

[70] Song YS, Kim MW, Moon C, Seo DJ, Han YS, Jo YH, et al. Extraction of chitin and chitosan from larval exuvium and whole body of edible meal worm, *Tenebrio molitor*. Entomology Research. 2018;**48**:227-233

[71] Bovera F, Marono S, Di Meo C, Piccolo G, Iannacconem F, Nizza A. Effect of mannanoligosaccharides supplementation on caecal microbial activity of rabbits. Animals. 2010;**4**:1522-1527. DOI: 10.1017/S1751731110000558

[72] Khempaka S, Chitsatchapong C, Molee W. Effect of chitin and protein constituents in shrimp head meal on growth performance, nutrient digestibility, intestinal microbial populations, volatile fatty acids and ammonia production in broilers. Journal of Applied Poultry Research. 2011;**20**:1-11

[73] Bovera F, Piccolo G, Gasco L, Marono S, Loponte R, Vassalotti G, et al. Yellow meal larvae (*Tennebrio molitor*) as a possible alternative to soybean meal in broiler diets. British Poultry Science. 2015;**56**(5):569-575. DOI: 10.1080/00071668.2015.1080815

[74] Loponte R, Nizza S, Bovera F, Riu ND. Growth performance, blood profiles and carcass triats of Barbarypatridges (Alectoris Barbara) fed two different insects larvae meals (*Tenebrio molitor* and *Hermetia illucens*). Research in Veterinary Science. 2017;**115**:2-6. DOI: 10.1016/j.rvsc.2017.04.017

[75] Benhabiles MS, Salah R, Lounici H, Drouiche N, Goosen MFA, Nameri N. Antibacterial activity of chitin, chitosan and its oligomers prepared from shrimp shell waste. Food Hydrocolloids. 2012;**29**:48-56

[76] Khoushab F, Yamabhai M. Chitin research revisited. Marine Drugs. 2010;**8**:1988-2012. DOI: 10.3390/md8071988

[77] Woods MJ, Cullere M, Emmenes LV, Vincenzi S, Pieterse E, Hoffman LC, et al. *Hermetia illucens* larvae reared on different substrates in broiler quail diets: Effect on apparent digestibility, feed-choice and growth performance. Journal of Insects as Food and Feed. 2019;**5**(2):89-98

[78] Bovera F, Loponte R, Marono S, Piccolo G, Parisi G, Laconisi V, et al. Use of *Tenebrio molitor* larvae meal as protein source in digestibility and carcass and meat traits. Journal of Animal Science. 2016;**94**:639-647

[79] Cutrignelli MI, Messina M, Tulli F, Randazzo B, Olivotto I, Gasco L. Evaluation of an insect meal of the Black Soldier Fly (*Hermetia illucens*) as soybean substitute: Intestinal morphometry, enzymatic and microbial activity in laying hens. Research in Veterinary Science. 2018;**117**:209-215. DOI: 10.1016/j.rvsc.2017.12.020

[80] De-Marco M, Martinez S, Hernandez F, Madrid J, Gai F, Rotolo L, et al. Nutritional value of two insect larval meals (*Tenebrio molitor* and *Hermetia illucens*) for broiler chickens: Apparent nutrient digestibility, apparent ileal amino acid digestibility and apparent metabolizable energy. Animal Feed Science and Technology. 2015;**209**:211-218

[81] Benzertiha A, Kieronczyk B, Rawski M, Jozefiak A, Kozlowski K, Jankowski J, et al. *Tenebrio molitor* and *Zophobas morio*. Full fat meals in broiler chicken diets: Effect on nutrient digestibility, digestive enzyme activities and cecal microbiome. Animals. 2019;**9**:1128. DOI: 10.3390/ani9721128

[82] Schiavone A, De Marco M, Rotolo L, Belforti M, Martinez Mir S, Madrid Sanche J, et al. Nutrient digestibility of *Hermetia illucens* and *Tenebrio molitor* meal in broiler chickens. In: Proc. 1st Int. Confer. Insects to Feed the World; Wageningen, The Netherlands. 2014. p. 73

[83] Van Huis A, Oonincx BGAB, Rojo S, Tomberlin JK. Insect as feed: House fly or black soldier fly. Journal of Insects as Food and Feed. 2020;**6**(3):221-229

[84] Rumpoid BA, Schluter OL. Potential and challenges of insect as an innovative source for food and feed production. Innovative Food Science and Emerging Technologies. 2013;**17**:1-11

[85] Bakuła T, Baranowski M, Czarnewicz A. The carcinogenic effects of benzoquinones produced by the flour beetle. Polish Journal of Veterinary Sciences. 2011;**14**:159-164

[86] Vandeweyer D, Milanovi'c V, Garofalo C, Osimani A, Clementi F, Van Campenhout L, et al. Real-time PCR detection and quantification of selected transferable antibiotic resistance genes in fresh edible insects from Belgium and the Netherlands. International Journal of Food Microbiology. 2019;**290**: 288-295

[87] Wynants E, Frooninckx L, Van Miert S, Geeraerd A, Claes J, Van Campenhout L. Risks related to the presence of *Salmonella* sp. during the rearing of mealworms (*Tenebrio molitor*) for food or feed: Survival in the substrate and transmission to the larvae. Food Control. 2019;**100**:227-234

[88] Van Broekhoven S, Gutierrez JM, De Rijk TC, De Nijs WC, Van Loon JJ. Degradation and excretion of the Fusarium toxin deoxynivalenol by an edible insect, the Yellow mealworm (*Tenebrio molitor* L.). World Mycotoxin Journal. 2017;**10**:163-169

[89] Van der Spiegel M, Noordam MY, Van der Fels-Klerx HJ. Safety of novel protein sources (insect, microalgae, seeweed, duck weed and rape seed) and legislative aspect of their application in food and food production. Comprehensive Reviews in Food Science and Food Safety. 2013;**12**:2-6. DOI: 10.1111/1541-4337.12032

[90] Schrogel P, Watjen W. Insects for food and feed safety aspects related to mycotoxins and metals. Review Foods. 2019;**8**:88. DOI: 10.3390/foods8080288

[91] Charlton AJ, Dickinson M, Wakefield ME, Fitches E, Kenis M, Han R, et al. Exploring the chemical safety of fly larvae as a source of protein for animal feed. Journal of Insects as Food and Feed. 2015;**1**:7-16

[92] Cai M, Hu R, Zhang K, Ma S, Zheng L, Yu Z, et al. Resistance of black soldier fly (Diptera: Stratiomyidae) larvae to combined heavy metals and potential application in municipal sewage sludge treatment. Environmental Science and Pollution Research. 2018;**25**:1559-1567

[93] Van Der Fels-Klerx HJ, Andriessen R, Van Schelt J, Van Dam R, De Rijk TC, Camenzuli L. Safety aspects when rearing insects for feed or food consumption. In: 69th Annual Meeting of the European Federation of Animal Science. Dubrovnic, Croatia: Wageningen Academic Publishers; 2018. pp. 27-31

[94] Purschke B, Scheibelberger R, Axmann S, Adler A, Jäger H. Impact of substrate contamination with mycotoxins, heavy metals and pesticides on the growth performance and composition of black soldier fly larvae (*Hermetia illucens*) for use in the feed and food value chain. Food Additives & Contaminants: Part A. 2017; **34**:1410-1420

[95] Schabel HG. Forest insects as food: A global review. In: Proceedings of a Workshop on Asia-Pacific Resources and their Potential for Development. United Kingdom: Taylor and Francis group; 2010. pp. 37-64

[96] Liu N, Abe M, Sabin LR, Hendriks GJ, Nagvi AS, Yu Z, et al. The exoribonuclease Nibbler controls 3′ end processing of microRNAs in Drosophila. Current Biology. 2011;**21**:1888-1893

[97] Jozefiak D, Engberg RM. Insects as poultry feed. In: Proc. 20th European Symposium on Poultry Nutrition. Czech Republic: World's Poultry Science Association; 2015. pp. 73-80

[98] Khusro M, Andrew NR, Nicholas A. Insects as poultry feed: A scoping study for poultry production systems in Australia. World's Poultry Science Journal. 2012;**68**:435-446

[99] Sánchez-Muros MJ, Barroso FG, Manzano-Agugliaro F. Insect meal as renewable source of food for animal feeding: A review. Journal of Cleaner Production. 2014;**65**:16-27

[100] Khan S, Khan RU, Sultan A, Khan M, Hayat SU, Shahid MS. Evaluation the suitability of maggot meal as a partial substitute of soya bean on the productive traits, digestibility indices and organoleptic properties of broiler meat. Journal of Animal Physiology and Animal Nutrition. 2016;**100**:649-656

[101] Kareem KY, Abdulla NR, Foo HL, Mohd AN, Zamri NS, Loh TC, et al. Effect of feeding larvae meal in the diets on growth performance, nutrient digestibility and meat quality in broiler chicken. The Indian Journal of Animal Sciences. 2018;**88**:180-1185

[102] Nguyen TT, Tomberlin JK, Vanlaerhoven S. Ability of black soldier fly (Diptera Stratiomyidae) larvae to recycle food waste. Environmental Entomology. 2015;**44**:406-410

[103] Nana P, Kimpara JM, Tiambo CK, Tiogue CT, Youmbi J, Choundong B, et al. Blacj soldier flies (*Hermetia illucens*) as recycles of organic waste and possible livestock. International Journal of Biological Sciences. 2018;**12**(5):2004-2015. DOI: 10.4314/ijbc.v12i5.4

[104] Van Huis A, Oonincx GAB. The environmental sustainability of insects as food and feed. A review. Agronomy for Sustainable Development. 2017;**37**:43

[105] Beskin KV, Holcomb CD, Cammack JA, Crippen TL, Knap AH, Sweet ST, et al. Larval digestion of different manure types by the black soldier fly (Diptera: Stratiomyidae) impacts associated volatile emissions. Waste Management. 2018;**74**:213-220

[106] Perednia DA, Anderson J, Rice A. A comparison of the greenhouse gas production of black soldier fly larvae versus aerobic microbial decomposition of an organic feed material. Research reviews. Journal of Ecology and Environmental Sciences. 2017;**5**:10-16

[107] Lalander CH, Fidjeland J, Diener S, Eriksson S, Vinneras B. High waste-to-biomass conversion and efficient *Salmonella* spp. reduction using black soldier fly for waste recycling. Agronomy for Sustainable Development. 2015;**35**(1):261-271. DOI: 10.1007/s13593-014-0235-4

[108] Gougbedji A, Agbohessou P, Laleye PA, Francis F, Medigo RC. Technical basis for the small scale production of black soldier fly *Hermetia illucens* (L. 1758) meal as fish feed in Benin. Journal of Agriculture and Food Research. 2021;**4**:100153. DOI: 10.1016/j.jafr.2021.100153

[109] World Wide Fund for nature (WWF). Beef, World Wild Fund for

Nature. Available from: https://www.worldwidelife.org/industries/beed.2019 [Accessed: November 2021]

[110] Jozefiak D, Józefiak A, Kieronczyk B, Rawski M, Świątkiewicz S, Długosz J, et al. Insects—A natural nutrient source for poultry—A review. Annals of Animal Science. 2016;**6**:297-313

[111] Kieronczyk B, Rawski M, Józefiak A, Mazurkiewicz J, Swiatkiewicz S, Siwek M, et al. Effects of replacing soybean oil with selected insect fats on broilers. Animal Feed Science and Technology. 2018; **240**:170-183

[112] Pastor B, Velasquez Y, Gobbi P, Rojo S. Conversion of organic wastes into fly larval biomass: Bottlenecks and challenges. Journal of Insects as Food and Feed. 2015;**1**:179-193

[113] Drew DJW, Pieterse E. Markets, money and maggots. Journal of Insects as Food and Feed. 2015;**1**:227-231

[114] Thevenot A, Rivera JL, Wilfart A, Maillard F, Hassouna M, Senga-Kiesse T, et al. Mealworm meal for animal feed: Environmental assessment and sensitivity analysis to guide future prospects. Journal of Cleaner Production. 2018;**170**:1260-1267

[115] Caruso D, Devic E, Subamia IW, Talamond P, Baras E. Technical Handbook of Domestication and Production of Diptera Black Soldier Fly (BSF) *Hermetia Illucens*, Stratiomyidae. Marseille, France: IRD Edition; 2015. pp. 30-38

[116] Dossey AT, Morales-Ramos JA, Guadalupe Rojas M, editors. Insects as Sustainable Food Ingredients: Production, Processing and Food Applications. Amsterdam, The Netherlands: Elsevier Inc.; 2016. pp. 153-201

[117] Cadinu LA, Borra P, Torre F, Delogu F, Madau FA. Insect rearing: Potential, challenges, and circulatory. Sustainability. 2020;**12**:4567

Chapter 4

Ruminal Microbiome Manipulation to Improve Fermentation Efficiency in Ruminants

Yosra Ahmed Soltan and Amlan Kumar Patra

Abstract

The rumen is an integrated dynamic microbial ecosystem composed of enormous populations of bacteria, protozoa, fungi, archaea, and bacteriophages. These microbes ferment feed organic matter consumed by ruminants to produce beneficial products such as microbial biomass and short-chain fatty acids, which form the major metabolic fuels for ruminants. The fermentation process also involves inefficient end product formation for both host animals and the environment, such as ammonia, methane, and carbon dioxide production. In typical conditions of ruminal fermentation, microbiota does not produce an optimal mixture of enzymes to maximize plant cell wall degradation or synthesize maximum microbial protein. Well-functioning rumen can be achieved through microbial manipulation by alteration of rumen microbiome composition to enhance specific beneficial fermentation pathways while minimizing or altering inefficient fermentation pathways. Therefore, manipulating ruminal fermentation is useful to improve feed conversion efficiency, animal productivity, and product quality. Understanding rumen microbial diversity and dynamics is crucial to maximize animal production efficiency and mitigate the emission of greenhouse gases from ruminants. This chapter discusses genetic and nongenetic rumen manipulation methods to achieve better rumen microbial fermentation including improvement of fibrolytic activity, inhibition of methanogenesis, prevention of acidosis, and balancing rumen ammonia concentration for optimal microbial protein synthesis.

Keywords: microbial manipulation, rumen, feed additives, phytochemicals, fiber degradation, microbial protein, acidosis

1. Introduction

Rumen inhabits several microbial populations, that is, bacteria, protozoa, fungi, bacteriophages, yeasts, and methanogens symbiotically, which are very dynamic, plastic, and redundant in function with the changes in diets though core microbiota persists, which has probably evolved by host-microbiota interaction in the evolutionary pressure over thousands of years [1]. A symbiotic relationship exists between rumen microbes and host animals in which both provide desirable substrates to each other mainly through these ways—1) physical breakdown of feed particles by mastication and rumination expands their surface area for microbial attachment and degradation, and consequently, microbes secrete various enzymes for dietary substrate degradation, 2) ruminal movements bring microbes in contact with the dietary substrate by mixing of digesta and consequently produce fermentation products (e.g., H_2, CO_2, ammonia, short-chain fatty acids (SCFAs), and 3) utilization (absorption and consumption) of the fermentation products for keeping optimal ruminal conditions (e.g., pH) to maintain microbial growth and microbial protein synthesis [2]. Therefore, due to the interactive ecosystem of the rumen, any modification to one component of this system has several effects on other components. The fermentation end products of any diet are incorporated into the final animal products (meat or milk). Thus, manipulation of the ruminal fermentation pathways is the most effective approach to improve ruminant health and production efficiency without exaggerated increases in nutrient supply. This in particular should help the small livestock holders in developing countries for continued production.

The literature explored various manipulation strategies including enhancing or inhibiting the growth or the metabolic activity of specific rumen microbiota (e.g., archaea for methanogenesis) and/or altering the ruminal fermentation toward specific pathways (e.g, decreasing H_2 production and increasing short-chain fatty acids (SCFAs) production [3, 4]. Extensive literature supports the supplementations of various rumen modifiers; however, efforts are still underway to find appropriate methods to simultaneously improve livestock production while reducing greenhouse effects on the environment. Through the following aspects, the most common methodologies for modifying the ruminal microbiome and fermentation characteristics are discussed in this chapter.

2. Enhancing fibrolytic activity and short-chain fatty acid production

Lignocellulose (complex polymers of cellulose, hemicellulose, pectin, and lignin) makes up the majority of the ruminant diet. Generally, forages, including crop residues, provide the main source of nutrition to ruminants that contribute to the food security and primary source of income of smallholder farmers in the developing countries [5–7]. This is also true where grazing animals are common in the developed countries. Hence, forage is virtually the only source of nutrition in the main beef-producing northern Australia, North and South America [8].

Although ruminants can digest fibrous feedstuffs, dietary cell wall polysaccharides are rarely completely degraded in the rumen. Less than 50% of the plant cell wall of most forage grasses are digested and utilized. This is attributed to the combination of the biochemical and physical barriers present in the ingested fibrous feedstuffs and retention time limitations of the ingested dietary substances in the rumen [9], resulting in excessive nutrient excretion, low nutrient intake, and a significant loss of dietary energy in the form of CH_4 emission [10]. Therefore, enhancing the rumen microbiota to degrade plant cell walls usually leads to improve animal productivity.

Ruminants cannot degrade lignocellulose themselves. An involved community of fibrolytic microorganisms catalyzes the degradation of the plant cell walls in the rumen. The major classical fibrolytic bacteria involved in fiber degradation are *Fibrobacter succinogenes, Ruminococcus albus, Ruminococcus flavefaciens, Butyrivibrio,* and *Prevotella* spp. [11]. Anaerobic fungi also contribute to degrade cell wall components and play a special role in degrading low-quality forages. Fungi are able to penetrate the plant tissue as a result of their filamentous growth and can degrade up to 34% of the lignin in plant tissues [12]. Fungi (i.e., *Neocallimastix* sp.) have a broad range of highly active fibrolytic enzymes and are the only known rumen microorganisms with exo-acting cellulose activity [11]. Cellulolytic activity is present in many rumen protozoa species, and the most efficient cellulose degraders are *Epidinium ecaudatum, Eudiplodinium maggii,* and *Ostracodinium dilobum* [13].

There are various well-established procedures that can be used to improve forage utilization including modifying ruminal microbial fermentation toward more fiber degradation. These include mechanical and chemical processing of forages and genetically engineering of plants for cell wall composition. However, we will focus on ruminal fibrolytic microorganisms and their products in the following sections of the chapter.

2.1 Genetically engineered fiber-degrading bacteria

The manipulation of genes in genetically engineered organisms can produce a product with novel specific characteristics that may have significant value. This concept was exploited in developing genetically modified fiber-degrading bacteria to optimize their activity by producing the correct mixture of fibrolytic enzymes to maximize plant cell wall degradation. *Ruminococcus* and *Fibrobacter* strains were the most targeted fiber-degrading bacteria for genetic modifications because they cannot produce exocellulases that are active against crystalline cellulose. Therefore, altering this activity would make them more potent [11]. The genome sequences of *F. succinogenes, R. albus,* and *Prevotella ruminicola* strains are available [11].

As early as 1995, Miyagi et al. [14] suggested that inoculation of genetically marked *R. albus* into a goat rumen might be of benefit to rumen function, but they found that the inoculant usually disappears from goat rumen after 14 days. One of the reasons for this is that bacteria reproduce within the physiological and ecological limits of the rumen ecosystem in which cooperative networks exist among ruminal microorganisms; since some organisms cleave specific bonds, others utilize particular substrates, while others produce inhibitors [11]. The scientists' sights were turned to *Butyrivibrio* species because they are among the most rumen bacteria capable of hemicellulose degradation and are regarded as being ecologically robust [15]. Gobius et al. [16] reported the successful transformation of a diverse range of eight strains of *Bu. fibrisolvens* with xylanase (family 10 glycosyl hydrolases) from rumen fungus *Neocallimastix patriciarum*. Glycosyl hydrolases family 10 was selected because it is different from family 11, which typically exists in *Bu. Fibrisolvens* and this family is characterized by high specific activity and resistance to proteolysis. The transformation was functionally successful and the *in vitro* fiber digestibility measurements revealed an improvement in plant fiber degradation by the recombinant xylanase; however, this still does not allow them to compete with the far more fibrolytic species *Fibrobacter* and *Ruminococcus* [11]. Another genetically engineered bacteria, *Bacteroides thetaiotaomicron* was inoculated at approximately 1% of the total population into *in vitro* dual-flow continuous culture fermenters and persisted for at least 144 h with relative abundances of 0.48–1.42% and increased fiber digestion, particularly hemicellulose fraction [17]. Generally, most of the experiments that used modified fibrolytic bacteria were *in vitro* trials. However, it should be taken into consideration that the *in vitro* fermenters did not express the full complement of rumen microorganisms (particularly protozoa). Moreover, this microbial manipulation application seems to be costly, especially for the small livestock holders in developing counties.

2.2 Direct-fed microbials

The concept of direct-fed microbials is different from the term probiotics. Probiotics were identified by any live microbial feed additive that may beneficially influence the host animals upon ingestion by improving microbial balance in the intestine [18]. Viable microbial communities, enzyme preparations, culture extracts, or combinations of those products were included in the concept of probiotic supplements [19]. The DFM has a narrower definition than probiotics as it is defined as a source of life, naturally occurring microorganisms alive, naturally occurring microorganisms that improve the digestive function of livestock. The DFM includes three main categories; bacterial, fungal, and a combination of both [20]. DFM must be alive to impact ruminal fermentation; thus, the viability and number of organisms fed must be ensured at the time of feeding. Lactic acid-producing and utilizing bacterial species of *Lactobacillus, Bifidobacterium, Streptococcus, Bacillus, Enterococcus, Propionibacterium*, *Megasphaera elsdenii* and *Prevotella bryantii,* and yeasts such as *Saccharomyces* and *Aspergillus* were the significant microbes of most of the DFM for livestock production [21].

DFM can grow under ruminal conditions and manipulate the microbial ecosystem. Various factors may affect the activity of DFM including microbial strains, time of feeding, feeding system, treatment period, physiological conditions, and dosages [20, 22]. The microbial strains seem to be the main influencer—DFM containing mainly lactic acid-producing and utilizing bacteria can manipulate the growth of microorganisms adapted to lactic acid in the rumen while preventing the drastic pH drops, for example, *M. elsdenii* [19]. DFM of *Propionibacterium* species can manipulate the fermentation pathways toward a more molar portion of propionate production [20, 23]. *Propionibacterium* is naturally found in high numbers in the rumen ecosystem and known to ferment lactate to propionate, providing more substrates for lactose synthesis in early lactation dairy cows, improving energy efficiency for the growing ruminants by reducing methane emission [20, 23].

Direct-fed microbials, based on fungal cultures, mainly contain *Saccharomyces cerevisiae* and *Aspergillus oryzae*, which can remove oxygen from the surfaces of freshly ingested feed particles to maintain the ruminal anaerobic conditions for the growth of cellulolytic bacteria [22, 24]. Moreover, the end metabolites of yeasts in the rumen can provide the ruminal microbiota with growth factors (i.e., rumen acetogens, digestive enzymes, anti-bacterial compounds, organic acids, and vitamins), resulting in stimulation of ruminal cellulolytic bacteria and maintenance of pH for optimal fiber degradation, and consequently greater production performance [21, 22]. Due to the low cost of DFM compared to other commercial feed additives, it can be included among the suitable solutions to manipulate the ruminal fiber degradation for the smallholder livestock sectors.

2.3 Exogenous fibrolytic enzymes

Products of exogenous fibrolytic enzymes (EFE) that contain primarily cellulolytic and xylanolytic activities can manipulate the ruminal fiber degradation, and improve feed conversion efficiency and thus lead to enhanced productive efficiency of ruminants [9]. Published literature suggests that the mode of actions of EFE products are likely different than that of DFM products. The activities introduced to the rumen by EFE are not novel to the ruminal ecosystem as they would act upon the same sites of the feed substrate particles as endogenous fibrolytic enzymes [25]. The release of reducing sugars by EFE is probably an essential mechanism by which EFE operates [26]. The degree of sugar release is dependent on the substrate types as well as the type of enzymes. The released sugars can attract secondary ruminal microbial colonization, or remove barriers to the microbial attachment to substrate feed particles by cleaving the linkage between phenolic compounds and polysaccharides [9]. As a result, the most significant effects of EFE probably occur in the interval between the arrival of the feed particles into the rumen and its colonization by ruminal microorganisms, as only the rate, not the extent, of cell wall degradation, has been improved [25]. EFE can also manipulate the rumen fibrolytic microorganisms by enhancing their endogenous fibrolytic activities.

Genes from ruminal fungi encoding cellulases, xylanases, mannanases, and endoglucanases have been successfully isolated. Protein bioengineering has been employed to improve the catalytic activity and substrate diversity of fibrolytic enzymes from ruminants. This has resulted in fibrolytic enzymes with up to 10 times higher specific activity, pH and temperature optima, and enhanced fiber-substrate binding activity than the original enzymes [27]. This, together with the low manufacturing cost, has led to more recent developments in the enzyme production industry, and as a result, a wide range of commercial EFE products is now available. Frequently the manufactures' recommended doses of most commercial EFE products have been measured under wide ranges of pH (4.2–6.5) and temperatures (40–57°C), which are not always close to typical ruminal conditions. Moreover, most of the commercial EFE products for ruminants are often referred to as xylanases or cellulases. However, none of these products comprise single enzymes; secondary enzyme activities are invariably present, namely, proteases, amylases, or pectinases [9]. A wide variety of feed substrates can be targeted by a single EFE product. Thus, the random addition of these products to ruminant diets without consideration for specific rumen conditions (pH 6.0–6.5 and 39°C) and the not yet tested efficiency for specific substrate will result in unpredictable effects and thus discouraging the adoption of the EFE technology [28, 29].

In general, enhancing the rumen microbiota to degrade the dietary fibers through the above-discussed strategies may lead to accelerating the energy production in the forms of short-chain fatty acids (SCFAs) and/or microbial protein synthesis. At the same time, it may also produce high amounts of CO_2 and CH_4.

3. Decreasing methanogenesis and increasing propionate production

The ruminal fermentation is the primary source of CH_4 emission from livestock; it is one of the most potent greenhouse gases featured by short atmospheric mean lifetime. Furthermore, a significant proportion of the ingested feed energy is also lost as CH_4 [40]. Methane is produced by methanogens mainly by reduction of CO_2 through the hydrogenotrophic pathway. Formic acid and methylamines produced by other ruminal bacteria are also reduced to CH_4 by some methanogens. Therefore, methanogens interact with other ruminal microorganisms (e.g., protozoa, bacteria, and fungi) through interspecies H_2 transfer [4]. Thus, maximizing metabolic H_2 flow away from CH_4 toward SCFAs production could improve production efficiency in ruminants and decrease environmental impact. There are various direct and indirect strategies to manipulate rumen methanogenesis; among these options, inhibiting the growth or the metabolic activity of methanogens seems to be the most effective approach. The efficiency of these strategies mainly depends on where methanogens reside. It can be seen from the smaller number of archaeal 16S rRNA gene sequences (461 vs. 8162) recovered from protozoa than from ruminal content or fluid [4]. Free methanogens are mainly integrated into the biofilm on the surfaces of feed particles where H_2-producing bacteria actively produce H_2. These methanogens protected by the biofilm may not be inhibited to an extent similar to the free-living peers by anti-methanogenic inhibitors [4]. Also, methanogens can be inhibited indirectly through inhibiting rumen ciliate protozoa. Based on fluorescence *in situ* hybridization analysis, about 16% of the rumen ciliate protozoa contained methanogens inside their cells [30]. Most rumen ciliate protozoa have hydrogenosomes, unique membrane-bound organelles producing H_2 by malate oxidization; therefore, these organelles can attract some species of methanogens as endosymbionts [4].

Methane formation pathways comprise of three main steps; transfer of methyl group to coenzyme M (CoM-SH), reduction of methyl-coenzyme M with coenzyme B (CoB-SH), and reusing heterodisulfide CoM-S-S-CoB [4, 31]. Thus, obstruction of any of these steps may manipulate CH_4 production. A wealth of literature on rumen CH_4 manipulation strategies in ruminants have been published recently, but relatively very few have emphasized the suitable mitigation strategies at the farm level [32]. Each method has some potential advantages and limitations. The principal interest for animal producers is income, as they usually do not take CH_4 mitigation strategies or climate changes into account. Thus, any strategy to mitigate greenhouse gasses emission would only be of practical interest if achievements on the efficiency of animal production can be obtained. This can be obtained through rumen CH_4 modifiers that enhance the production of SCFAs and/or reduce proteases. The following part addresses some of these microbial modifiers.

3.1 Ionophores

Ionophores are polyether antibiotics that act as inhibitors to hydrogen-producing bacteria. They are widely used as successful growth promoters in the livestock industry due to their ability to modulate rumen fermentation toward propionate production, thereby decreasing CH_4 production. Since propionate and CH_4 are terminal acceptors for metabolic H_2, any increase in propionate production may accompany reduced CH_4. In addition, ionophores positively affect ruminal fermentation through inhibition of deamination compared to proteolysis, inhibition of hydrolysis of triglycerides, and biohydrogenation of unsaturated fatty acids, while enhancing the trans-octadecenoic isomers (cited from [33]).

From the literature, monensin and lasalocid are the most well-known ionophore-type antimicrobials used as rumen modifiers. Mainly, they inhibit Gram-positive bacteria; however, they can also inhibit some Gram-negative bacteria. Ionophores decrease CH_4 production by inhibiting H_2 producing bacteria by penetrating the bacterial cell wall membrane. They act as H^+/Na^+ and H^+/K^+ antiporters, dissipating ion gradients required for the synthesis of ATP, transport of nutrients, and other essential cellular activities in bacteria, resulting in retardation of cell growth and cell death [4, 34]. Monensin can decrease total methanogens number in cattle, and also alter the community composition of methanogen species, for example, monensin decreased the population of *Methanomicrobium* spp. while increasing that of *Methanobrevibacters* spp. [4].

Unfortunately, ionophores present a temporary impact on ruminal manipulation effects due to the adaptation of the microorganisms of these inhibitors. Ionophores are now restricted due to the possible resistance of pathogenic microorganisms to antibiotics [33]. Recently, the global scenario has shifted the interest toward plant natural feed additives with potential abilities to modulate CH_4 emission [35, 36]. Moreover, the type of the dietary feeds affects the efficiency of ionophores with the better effect of ionophores observed in high starch diets [33]. Thus, this approach seems to be less effective for the small livestock holders in most developing countries since the forages are the main ingredient in the diets.

3.2 Natural feed additives as rumen modifiers

3.2.1 Plant secondary compounds

Numerous plant secondary compounds (PSC), including tannins, flavonoids, saponins, essential oils (EOs), organosulfur compounds, have been recognized as having the potential to modulate ruminal microbial fermentation [37–39]. Plant secondary compounds are natural phytochemicals with the potential ability to manipulate rumen fermentation without causing microbial resistance or residual noxious effects on animal products [3]. Unlike ionophores, the different active components found in plant extracts may manipulate ruminal microbiota through more potent mechanisms of action (e.g., antimicrobial and antioxidant), which may avoid the risk of losing activity over time [40].

3.2.2 Tannins

Tannins are polyphenolic compounds with different molecular weights ranging from 500 to 5000 Da [41]. Tannins are classified into two major groups, that is, condensed (CT) and hydrolyzable tannins (HT). CT are proanthocyanidins consisting of oligomers or polymers of flavan-3-ol subunits. They act through binding with dietary proteins and carbohydrates by making strong complexes at ruminal pH [41–43]. Therefore, they are the most plant secondary metabolites studied in terms of rumen modulation pathways.

The literature reported quite various effects of CT supplementations regarding CH_4 mitigation [38]. Some studies suggest a direct effect of CT on methanogens by binding with the proteinaceous adhesin or parts of the cell envelope, which impairs the establishment of methanogens-protozoa complex and decreases interspecies H_2 transfer, and inhibits growth [44]. Other studies suggest an indirect effect of CT through the anti-protozoal effect. However, the effects of CT on rumen protozoal activity are varied in the literature, probably because some of the CTs have a direct effect on rumen methanogenic archaea, which are not associated with the protozoa. Tannins also can indirectly inhibit CH_4 per unit of the animal product through tannin–protein or organic matter complexes under ruminal conditions, while protein from these complexes is released post ruminally, making it available for gastric digestion at abomasum and small intestine conditions, leading to enhancing the animal productivity [43]. Another theory is that tannins can act as H_2 sink reducing the availability of H_2 for CO_2 reduction to CH_4, implying that 1.2 mol CH_4 is produced per mol of catechin [44].

Tree foliages are good feed resources for the small ruminants, which are rich in protein and perform catalytic functions in improving ruminal fermentation, especially in low-quality forage-based diets in developing countries [45]. The nutritionists have paid great attention to the tanniferous legumes and tree foliages as alternative cheap feed resources (especially in drought conditions and arid and semi-arid regions) and to achieve CH_4 mitigation goals in the developing countries [46]. Many plants were investigated in the literature; however, the results are highly variable among studies. Soltan et al. [43] studied various tanniniferous browsers and found that some plants (i.e., *Prosopis* and *Leucaena*) similarly modulate ruminal fermentation as ionophores perform by decreasing the acetate to propionate ratio, CH_4 and NH_3-N, while *Acacia* reduced CH_4 through decreasing fiber degradation although it had similar CT concentration as *Leucaena*. Thus, it seems that not only does tannin concentration play a role in the modulation of the ruminal fermentation process, but also types, molecular weights are important in determining tannin potency in modulating rumen fermentation patterns. The presence of HT and other plant secondary metabolites (mimosine in *Leucaena*) together with CT can interact with the action of CT [44, 47].

3.2.3 Saponins

Saponins are a group of plant secondary metabolites with high molecular weight glycosides in which a sugar is linked to a hydrophobic aglycone. It can be generally classified as steroidal and triterpenoid [48, 49]. The effects of saponins on rumen fermentation modulation have been reviewed extensively [49]. The main biological effect of saponins is on the cell membranes of bacteria and protozoa. Saponins are highly toxic to protozoa compared with bacteria because saponins can form complexes with sterols present in the protozoal membrane surface, disrupting the membrane function [49]. Thus, it can indirectly affect the methanogenic archaea through their symbiotic relationship with rumen protozoa [38]. However, some literature assumed that the effects of saponins on rumen protozoa could be transient due to the ability of ruminal bacteria to degrade saponins into sapogenins. The sapogenin compound cannot affect protozoa [50].

3.2.4 Essential oils

Essential oils (EO) are volatile aromatic complexes obtained from different plant volatile fractions by steam distillation. They can be obtained from various plant parts including leaf, stem, fruit, root, seed, flower, bark, and petal. EO contains numerous bioactive substances; the most important ones are terpenoids (monoterpenoids and sesquiterpenoids) and phenylpropanoids. Due to the lipophilic properties of these components, EO act against various rumen bacteria through interacting with the cell membrane [3].

Several EO compounds, either in pure form or in mixtures, had antioxidant and anti-bacterial properties; therefore, they can modulate the ruminal fermentation pathways [51]. The EO, unlike ionophores, does not alter the ruminal microbial activities through a specific mode of action. Therefore, EO may have more potent mechanisms of action that may not likely lose their effectiveness over time. Soltan et al. [40] suggested two mechanisms in explaining how combination of phenylpropanes and terpene hydrocarbons components in EO mixtures work together to enhance additive antimicrobial activity—1) phenolic compounds may increase cell membrane permeability through the action of hydroxyl group, thus facilitating the transport of terpene hydrocarbons into the microbial cells, which then combine with proteins and enzymes inside the cells; 2) phenolic compounds could increase the size, number or duration of the existence of the pores created by the binding of terpene hydrocarbons with proteins in cell membranes.

The effects of EO on rumen fermentation are variable depending on concentrations, types, diet and adaptation period, but most EO are found to have anti-methanogenic properties [35, 52]. Patra and Yu [52] studied various EO with different chemical structures (clove, eucalyptus, origanum, peppermint, and garlic oil) *in vitro* at three different concentrations (0.25, 0.50, and 1.0 g/L) for their effect on CH_4 production and archaeal abundance and diversity and they found that all these EO suppressed CH_4 production, but the extent of CH_4 inhibition and ruminal fermentation differed among the EO. Further studies are needed to understand the interactions of the active compounds with the dietary ingredients and their activity against specific methanogens should be identified without adverse effects on fermentation patterns and rumen fiber degradability, as well as the different doses for each EO. Also, attention needs to be paid to the palatability as some EO may adversely affect palatability and dry matter intake due to the aroma they add to the ration. Therefore, many products of encapsulated EO are available in commercial forms, but this raises the question of the suitability of these products as feed additives at the farm level in developing countries.

3.2.5 Propolis

Propolis is a mixture of resinous substances collected from buds of deciduous trees and crevices in the bark of coniferous and deciduous trees and secretions by honeybees [53, 54]. The bees use propolis to fill cracks, cover hive walls and embalm invading intruder insects or small animals [55, 56]. The literature reported that the chemical composition of propolis is highly variable by bee collection site since geographical location plays an important role [54]. The most bioactive components are belonging to groups of isoflavones, flavonoids, and fatty acids that have been reported to be biologically active [53]. Recently, bee propolis has been recognized as a natural alternative feed additive to antibiotics in ruminant diets [54]. Compared to ionophores (e.g., monensin), different propolis sources can reduce CH_4 production while improving the organic matter digestibility and total SCFAs *in vitro* and *in vivo* [53, 57]. Morsy et al. [58] reported that CH_4 reduction caused by propolis supplementation is accompanied by increasing urinary allantoin, total purine derivatives, and enhancements of individual and total SCFAs. Thus, they suggested that propolis can help in the redirection of ruminal organic matter degradation from CH_4 production to microbial synthesis and SCFAs. From a practical view, propolis can be a promising feed additive in the vegetation places where it is produced in a large amount such as Brazil.

3.3 Plant oils

Fats are usually used as energy sources for dairy cattle. The addition of fats is a promising approach for modulating rumen microbial communities and the fermentation process. Fats are known to inhibit microbial activity; however, supplementing fats up to 6% of dry matter has shown no adverse effects on total nutrient digestibility and total SCFAs [59]. A meta-analysis study suggests that methane emissions can be declined by 0.66 g/kg DM intake with each percentage increase in dietary fats, within dietary fat concentrations of 1.24–11.4% [59]. Fats containing high levels of C12:0, C18:3, and polyunsaturated fatty acids up to 6% of the dietary diet may be considered for CH_4 mitigation without compromising the productivity in dairy cattle [59].

Plant oil supplements can modulate CH_4 directly by inhibiting rumen protozoa and methanogens while enhancing biohydrogenation of polyunsaturated fatty acids (PUFA) to act as ruminal hydrogen sink for hydrogen produced by rumen microorganisms and reducing fiber degradation with less H_2 production in the rumen [60]. The literature showed variable effects of plant oils on CH_4 emission and rumen fermentation; this might be related to the oil type (free oil or whole seed), diet composition (forage to-concentrate ratio), and fatty acid type (short-chain or PUFA) present in diets [59]. Generally, consideration of vegetable oils supplementation to lower CH_4 emission may depend upon the cost and expected outcome effect on animal productivity.

3.4 Chitosan

Chitosan is a natural polycationic polymer, nontoxic, biocompatible, biodegradable; thus, it is safe for human as well as animal consumption [61]. It is a linear polysaccharide composed of two repeated units—D-glucosamine and N-acetyl-D-glucosamine linked by β-(1–4)-linkages [61]. It can be found in the structural exoskeleton of insects, crustaceans, mollusks, cell walls of fungi, and certain algae, but it is mainly obtained from marine crustaceans [62]. It is characterized by anti-inflammatory, antitumor, antioxidative, anticholesterolemic, hemostatic, and analgesic effects. Moreover, it has a high antimicrobial affinity against a wide range of bacteria, fungi, and protozoa; therefore, it has been recently tested as a rumen fermentation modulator and considered as a promising natural agent with CH_4 mitigating effects [61]. The antimicrobial mechanism of chitosan can include interactions at the cell surface and outer membranes through electrostatic forces, the replacement of Ca^{+2} and Mg^{+2} ions, the destabilization of the cell membrane, and leakage of intracellular substances, and cell death. The antimicrobial properties of chitosan can also include chelating capacity for various metal ions and the inhibition of mRNA and protein synthesis [61].

It seems chitosan activity depends on the diet type as well as the ruminal pH. The literature reports suggest that the maximum effect of chitosan is noted when grain (starch) is incorporated in the ration at low pH values, shifting the fermentation pattern to a more propionate production pathway, which could be explained by the higher sensitivity of Gram-positive bacteria than Gram-negative bacteria against chitosan [61, 63]. This type of change in ruminal fermentation by chitosan results in reductions in CH_4 production. Moreover, supplementation of chitosan alters the rumen bacterial communities related to fatty acids biohydrogenation, that is, *Butyrivibrio* group and *Butyrivibrio proteoclasticus* that lead to increases in concentrations of milk unsaturated fatty acids and cis-9,trans-11 conjugated linoleic acid [64].

3.5 Chemical feed additives

Numerous chemical additives were used to modulate the rumen microbial activity for optimizing animal productivity, namely, defaunating agents, and anti-methanogenic agents to reduce CH_4 emission. Patra et al. [4] reported the most promising anti-methanogenic agents that effectively lower CH_4 without adverse effects on rumen degradability or producing SCFAs and each of which works through different modes of action when added together to additively decrease CH_4 production. These include halogenated sulfonated compounds (e.g., 2-bromoethanesulfonate, 2-chloroethanesulfonate, and 3-bromopropanesulfonate), 3-nitrooxypropanol (3NOP), nitrate, and ethyl-3NOP are used to inhibit methyl-CoM reductase activity, the final limiting step to complete the methanogenesis pathways. Halogenated aliphatic compounds with 1 or 2 carbons can impair the corrinoid enzymes function and inhibit cobamide-dependent methyl group transfer in methanogenesis or may serve as terminal electron (e^-) acceptors. Some agents, namely, lovastatin and mevastatin were found to inhibit 3-hydroxy-3-methylglutaryl coenzyme, which is essential in the mevalonate pathway to form isoprenoid alcohols of methanogen cell membranes [4]. The addition of nitrate has two benefits—it can inhibit methanogenesis and acts as a nonprotein nitrogen source, which could be useful in low-quality base diets [65].

4. Control of acidosis

Diets containing high amounts of rapidly fermenting soluble carbohydrate result in pH drop due to excessive production of lactate or VFA or a combination of both, which may be of subacute ruminal acidosis (pH between 5.0 to 5.5) or acute acidosis (<5.0) type with acute or chronic in duration [66]. The consequences of acidosis range widely along with death and more importantly lower productivity, especially in subacute ruminal acidosis [66, 67]. Decreasing the ruminal pH leads to inhibition of rumen cellulolytic bacteria. Therefore, maintaining ruminal pH at the average level (5.8–7.2) is an essential factor to balance the rumen microorganisms between acid producers and consumers. In this context, buffering reagents and alkalizer (e.g., sodium bicarbonate, magnesium oxide, and calcium magnesium carbonate), direct-fed microbials, and malate supplementation may increase pH in the rumen and production when ruminants are fed with high-grain based diets [66, 68]. Malate supplementation can stimulate Selenomonas ruminantium that converts lactate to VFA [69]. Marden et al. [70] reported that the inclusion of 150 g of sodium bicarbonate increased total ruminal VFA concentration by 11.7% compared to the control diet fed to lactating cows. The addition of sodium bicarbonate, magnesium oxide, and calcium magnesium carbonate reduced the duration of time ruminal pH persisted below 5.8 in lactating dairy cows fed a high-starch (342 g/kg DM) containing diet and increased milk and fat yield, and milk fat concentration, but reduced milk *trans*-fatty acids isomers [71]. The efficacy of the acid-neutralizing capacity of the alkalizers depends upon physical and chemical properties that influence the solubility in the ruminal conditions. However, in developing country conditions, the acidosis problems are usually less severe as ruminants are mostly fed with roughage-based diets.

5. Enhancing ruminal microbial protein synthesis

Microbial protein in the rumen (RMP) accounts for between 50 and 90% of the protein entering into the duodenum and supplies the majority of the amino acids required for growth and milk protein synthesis [72]. Therefore, increasing RMP synthesis is important for improving animal productivity. Moreover, increasing the RMPS is an effective strategy to decrease protein (i.e., nitrogen) excretion in livestock since the dietary protein unless utilized properly by ruminal microorganisms is degraded to ammonia in the rumen, and ammonia is absorbed from the rumen, metabolized to urea in the liver, and excreted in urine causing environmental nitrogen pollution [10, 73].

There are many factors affecting RMP synthesis including dry matter intake, type of the ration fed (forage to concentrate ratio), the flow rate of digesta in the rumen, the sources, and synchronization of nitrogen and energy sources [74]. Among these, the amount of energy supplied to rumen microbes was found to be the main factor affecting the amount of nitrogen incorporated into RMP. Phosphorylation at the substrate level and electron transport level are two significant mechanisms of energy generation within microbial cells [75]. Based on 10 reconstructed pathways associated with the energy metabolism in the ruminal microbiome, Lu et al. [75] found that the energy-rich diet increased the total abundance of substrate-level phosphorylation enzymes in the glucose fermentation and F-type ATPase of the electron transporter chain more than the protein-rich diet. Therefore, they concluded that energy intake induces higher RMP yield more than protein intake. In this context, any factor affecting the available amount of soluble carbohydrates to rumen microbes will affect the efficiencies of RMP synthesis. Therefore, most of the previously mentioned rumen modifiers (e.g., plant secondary metabolites, dietary oil) may affect the RMP synthesis; however, most of the studies have ignored the determination of RMP.

Maximizing RMP synthesis seems to be the most effective approach for the small livestock holders in most developing countries since microbial protein sometimes becomes the only protein source for the animals fed on poor quality forage diets with low or without concentrate supplementations. Balancing the diets of these animals by supplementing of leaves of legumes, urea-molasses multinutrient blocks, urea in the form of slow ammonia release, and other nonprotein nitrogen resources found to be favorable for RMP synthesis [8, 10, 29, 73]. It has been recognized that feeding high true proteins (the most expensive ingredients in the ruminant diet) can be utilized by ruminal bacteria in about the same way as the ammonia from nonprotein nitrogen (e.g., urea). The optimum concentrations of ammonia in the rumen for maximal RMP synthesis are about 50–60 mg/L and 27–133 mg/L from the *in vitro* and *in vivo* studies, respectively [73].

Reduction in CH_4 production can enhance the RMP synthesis. Soltan et al. [10, 29] observed that inclusion of *Leucaena* in sheep diet up to 35% with or without polyethylene glycol enhanced the RMP and the body nitrogen retention while reducing CH_4 emission; they suggested that optimizing microbial growth efficiency might help to redirect organic matter degraded from CH_4 formation to RMP synthesis. Plants or feed additives containing phytochemicals with high antioxidant activity can promote more nutrients for microbial uptake, enhancing RMP synthesis, while reducing CH_4 emission due to lessening the ruminal oxidative stress [36, 53].

6. Reduction of ruminal protein degradation and ammonia production

From an economic view, dietary protein concentrates increase production costs, especially for developing countries. Furthermore, the microbial population in the rumen has a high proteolytic capacity to degrade the dietary protein. Therefore, nutritionists are interested in formulating diets with ruminal undegradable protein sources. The protein degradation in rumen depends mainly on three processes—proteolysis, peptidolysis, and deamination. Many protein-degrading bacteria are naturally found under ruminal conditions, that is, *Ruminobacter amylophilus*, *P. ruminicola*, *Butyrivibrio fibrisolvens, S. ruminantium*, *Streptococcus bovis*, and *P. bryantii*. There are many amino acid-fermenting bacteria, that is, *Clostridium sticklandii*, *Clostridium aminophilum*, *M. elsdenii*, *B. fibrisolvens, P. ruminicola, S. bovis,* and *S. ruminantium* [73]. Increased ruminal ammonia concentration is an indicator of the high degradation of dietary protein. Many factors can affect ruminal protein degradation and ammonia concentration, such as the type of dietary protein, the energy sources, the predominant microbial population, the rumen passage rate, rumen pH [35]. The ruminal bacteria can utilize ammonia for the synthesis of amino acids required for their growth. The optimal ammonia concentration needed to maximize the RMP synthesis ranges from 88 to 133 mg/L [76].

Several inhibitors of ruminal microbial protein degradation and ammonia production were reported in the literature. Condensed tannins, slow-release urea products, encapsulated nitrate, clays (e.g., bentonite and zeolite that acts through cation exchange capacity), and biochar were found to reduce the rapid increase in ammonia production and maintained the ruminal pH. Urea pool in the rumen is contributed from urea in the diet and recycling of urea through saliva and ruminal wall. The urease enzyme produced by the ruminal microbiota rapidly degrades urea to ammonia causing ammonia toxicity and inefficient urea utilization when used in excessive amounts [73]. Inhibitors of urease may reduce the risk of ammonia toxicity and efficient utilization of urea and other nonprotein nitrogen compounds [77].

7. Enhancing functional values of milk and meat

Ruminant-derived foods (milk and meat) contain a high amount of saturated fatty acids, which are associated with human health concerns. Therefore, improving the functional value of ruminants' products by increasing the content of beneficial fatty acids (FAs) and decreasing detrimental ones, specifically, decreasing the content of saturated FAs and increasing n-3 FAs and conjugated linoleic acids (e.g., cis-9, trans-11 C18:2, also called rumenic acid) have been great interests among the researchers [78]. Manipulating ruminal biohydrogenation of polyunsaturated fatty acids (PUFAs) has been the target to increase meat and milk content of rumenic acid and vaccenic acid, as both compounds are major intermediates in the biohydrogenation. To elevate rumenic acid content in products, inhibiting the last step of biohydrogenation needs to be attempted without affecting lipolysis and isomerization and reduction of linoleic acid and linolenic acid to rumenic acid and vaccenic acid. Alternatively, to elevate PUFAs in meat and milk, in particular n-3FAs, inhibition of early steps of biohydogenation should be targeted. Secondary compounds such as tannins, saponins, or essential oils rich in terpenes present in plants and forages or supplementation of vegetable oil can improve some aspects of meat and milk quality including n-3 FAs, conjugated linoleic acids, antioxidant properties [73, 79–81].

8. Conclusions

The ruminal fermentation end products are typically the outputs of several interactive reactions among the rumen microbial populations. Manipulations of rumen microbial fermentation toward enhancing fiber digestibility, SCFAs production, and outflow of microbial biomass, while reducing ammonia and CH_4 emission are the most probable ways to improve animal productivity. Numerous rumen fermentation modifiers have been studied during the last few decades; however, their positive effects are sometimes associated with undesirable effects or highly significant costs (e.g., ionophore antibiotics, anti-methanogenic chemical feed additives, or essential oils). Moreover, most of these modifiers exhibited inconsistent efficacy in the literature mainly because of the variability in animal age, breed, diet formulation, physiological status, rumen microbial resistance, and adaptation. Despite the long history of studies on the rumen modifiers, most of the measurements are determined through the treatment period but knowledge is still limited on animal responses in later life or impacts on human health and growth. However, there is unanimous agreement that an ample array of drought-tolerant plants containing effective bioactive compounds, DFM, fibrolytic enzymes, and nonprotein nitrogen sources would cost-effectively modify the ruminal fermentation. Therefore, a combination of two or more of these rumen modifiers with complementary modes of action may be a promising approach to optimize the productivity of ruminants in developing countries.

Conflict of interest

The authors declare no conflict of interest.

Author details

Yosra Ahmed Soltan[1] and Amlan Kumar Patra[2*]

1 Faculty of Agriculture, Department of Animal and Fish Production, Alexandria University, Alexandria, Egypt

2 Department of Animal Nutrition, West Bengal University of Animal and Fishery Sciences, Kolkata, India

*Address all correspondence to: patra_amlan@yahoo.com

References

[1] Patra AK. Characteristics of ruminal microbial community: Evolutionary and ecological perspectives. Indian Journal of Animal. Health. 2020;**59**(Special 2):114-127

[2] Belanche A, Patra AK, Morgavi DP, Suen G, Newbold CJ, Yáñez-Ruiz DR. Editorial: Gut microbiome modulation in ruminants: Enhancing advantages and minimizing drawbacks. Frontiers in Microbiology. 2021;**11**:622002

[3] Calsamiglia S, Busquet M, Cardozo PW, Castillejos L, Ferret A. Essential oils as modifiers of rumen microbial fermentation: Invited review. Journal of Dairy Science. 2007;**90**:2580-2595

[4] Patra A, Park T, Kim M, Yu Z. Rumen methanogens and mitigation of methane emission by anti-methanogenic compounds and substances. Journal of Animal Science and Biotechnology. 2017;**8**:13

[5] Salama HSA, El-Zaiat HM, Sallam SMA, Soltan YA. Agronomic and qualitative characterization of multi-cut berseem clover (*Trifolium alexandrinum* L.) cultivars. Journal of the Science of Food and Agriculture. 2020;**100**:3857-3865

[6] Singh P, Hundal JS, Patra AK, Wadhwa M, Sharma A. Sustainable utilization of *Aloe vera* waste in the diet of lactating cows for improvement of milk production performance and reduction of carbon footprint. Journal of Cleaner Production. 2021;**288**:125118. DOI: 10.1016/j.jclepro.2020.125118

[7] Soltan Y, Filho AA, Abdalla A, Schiavinatto P, Costa C. Replacing maize with low tannin sorghum grains: lamb growth performance, microbial protein synthesis and enteric methane production. Animal Production Science. 2021;**61**:1348-1355. DOI: 10.1071/AN20605

[8] Wadhwa M, Bakshi MPS, Makkar HPS. Modifying gut microbiomes in large ruminants: Opportunities in non-intensive husbandry systems. Animal Frontiers. 2016;**6**:27-36

[9] Wang Y, McAllister TA. Rumen microbes, enzymes and feed digestion-a review. Asian-Australasian Journal of Animal Sciences. 2002;**15**:1659-1676

[10] Soltan YA, Morsy AS, Sallam SMA, Lucas RC, Louvandini H, Kreuzer M, et al. Contribution of condensed tannins and mimosine to the methane mitigation caused by feeding *Leucaena leucocephala*. Archives of Animal Nutrition. 2013a;**67**:169-184

[11] Krause DO, Denman SE, Mackie RI, Morrison M, Rae AL, Attwood GT, et al. Opportunities to improve fiber degradation in the rumen: microbiology, ecology, and genomics. FEMS Microbiology Reviews. 2003;**27**:663-693

[12] McSweeney CS, Dulieu A, Katayama Y, Lowry JB. Solubilisation of lignin by the ruminal anaerobic fungus Neocallimastixpatriciarum. Applied and Environmental Microbiology. 1994;**60**:2985-2989

[13] Dehority BA. Rumen Microbiology. Nottingham: Nottingham University Press; 2003

[14] Miyagi T, Kaneichi K, Aminov RI, Kobayashi Y, Sakka K, Hoshino S, et al. Enumeration of transconjugated Ruminococcusalbus and its survival in the goat rumen ecosystem. Applied and Environmental Microbiology. 1995;**61**:2030-2032

[15] Weimer PJ. Why don't ruminal bacteria digest cellulose faster? Journal of Dairy Science. 1996;**79**:1496-1502

[16] Gobius KS, Xue GP, Aylward JH, Dalrymple BP, Swadling YJ,

McSweeney CS, et al. Transfromation and expression of an anaerobic fungal xylanase in several strains of the rumen bacterium *Butyrivibrio fbrisolvens*. Journal of Applied Microbiology. 2002;**93**:122-133

[17] Ziemer CJ, Sharp R, Stern MD, Cotta MA, Whitehead TR, Stahl DA. Persistence and functional impact of a microbial inoculant on native microbial community structure, nutrient digestion and fermentation characteristics in a rumen model. Systemic and Applied Microbiology. 2002;**25**:416-422

[18] Mahesh MS, Mohanta RK, Patra AK. Probiotics in livestock and poultry nutrition and health. In: Goel G, Kumar A, editors. Advances in Probiotics for Sustainable Food and Medicine. Microorganisms for Sustainability. Vol. volume 21. Singapore: Springer; 2021. pp. 149-179

[19] Yoon IK, Stern MD. Influence of direct-fed microbials on ruminal microbial fermentation and performance of ruminants: A review. Asian-Australasian Journal of Animal Sciences. 1995;**8**:533-555

[20] Elghandour MY, Salem AZM, Castañeda JSM, Camacho LM, Kholif AE, Chagoyán JCV. Direct-fed microbes: A tool for improving the utilization of low quality roughages in ruminants. Journal of Integrative Agriculture. 2015;**14**:526-533

[21] Seo JK, Kim SW, Kim MH, Upadhaya SD, Kam DK, Ha JK. Direct-fed microbials for ruminant animals. Asian-Australasian Journal of Animal Sciences. 2010;**23**:1657-1667

[22] Patra AK. The use of live yeast products as microbial feed additives in ruminant nutrition. Asian Journal of Animal and Veterinary Advannces. 2012;**7**:366-375

[23] Vyas D, McGeough EJ, Mohammed R, McGinn SM, McAllister TA, Beauchemin KA. Effects of *Propionibacterium* strains on ruminal fermentation, nutrient digestibility and methane emissions in beef cattle fed a corn grain finishing diet. Animal. 2014;**8**:1807-1815

[24] Newbold CJ, Wallace RJ, McIntosh FM. Mode of action of the yeast Saccharomyces cerevisiaeas a feed additive for ruminants. British Journal of Nutrition. 1996;**76**:249-261

[25] McAllister TA, Hristov AN, Beauchemin KA, RodeL M, Cheng KJ. Enzymes in ruminant diets. In: Bedford MR, Partridge GG, editors. Enzymes in Farm Animal Nutrition. CABI Publishing, CAB International: UK; 2001. pp. 273-298

[26] Beauchemin KA, Rode LM. Use of feed enzymes inruminant nutrition. In: Rode LM, editor. Animal Science Research and Development Meeting Future Challenges. Minister of Supply and Services: Ottawa, Canada; 1996. pp. 103-131

[27] Selinger LB, Forsberg CW, Cheng KJ. The rumen: a unique source of enzymes for enhancing livestock production. Anaerobe. 1996;**2**:263-284

[28] Beauchemin KA, Colombatto D, Morgavi DP, Yang WZ. Use of exogenous fibrolytic enzymes to improve feed utilization by ruminants. Journal of Animal Science. 2003;**81**:37-47

[29] Soltan YA, Abdalla AL, Silva LRF, Natel AS, Morsy AS, Louvandini H. Response of different tropical pasture grass species to treatment with fibrolytic enzymes in terms of in vitro ruminal nutrient degradation and methanogenesis. Animal Nutrition and Feed Technology. 2013b;**13**:551-568

[30] Lloyd D, Williams AG, Amann R, Hayes AJ, Durrant L, Ralphs JR. Intracellular prokaryotes in rumen

ciliate protozoa: Detection by confocal laser scanning microscopy after in situ hybridization with fluorescent 16S rRNA probes. European Journal of Protistology. 1996;**32**:523-531

[31] Tapio I, Snelling TJ, Strozzi F, Wallace RJ. The ruminal microbiome associated with methane emissions from ruminant livestock. Journal of Animal Science and Biotechnology. 2017;**8**:7-17

[32] Ku-Vera JC, Castelán-Ortega OA, Galindo-Maldonado FA, Arango J, Chirinda N, Jiménez-Ocampo R, et al. Strategies for enteric methane mitigation in cattle fed tropical forages. Review: Animal. 2020a;**14**:s453-s463. DOI: 10.1017/S1751731120001780

[33] McGuffey RK. A 100-year review: Metabolic modifiers in dairy cattle nutrition. Journal of Dairy Science. 2017;**100**:10113-10142

[34] Tedeschi LO, Fox DG, Tylutki TP. Potential environmental benefits of ionophores in ruminant diets. Journal of Environmental Quality. 2003;**32**:1591-1602

[35] Patra AK, Yu Z. Effects of Adaptation of in vitro rumen culture to garlic oil, nitrate, and saponin and their combinations on methanogenesis, fermentation, and abundances and diversity of microbial populations. Frontiers in Microbiology. 2015;**6**:1434

[36] Soltan YA, Hashem NM, Morsy AS, El-Azrak KM, Nour El-Din A, Sallam SM. Comparative effects of *Moringa oleifera* root bark and monensin supplementations on ruminal fermentation, nutrient digestibility and growth performance of growing lambs. Animal Feed Science and Technology. 2018a;**235**:189-201

[37] Kholif AE, Anele UY, Patra AK, Varadyova Z. Editorial: The use of phytogenic feed additives to enhance productivity and health in ruminants. Frontiers in Veterinary Science. 2021;**8**:685262

[38] Patra AK, Saxena J. A new perspective on the use of plant secondary metabolites to inhibit methanogenesis in the rumen. Phytochemistry. 2010;**71**:1198-1122

[39] Patra AK. Recent advances in measurement and dietary mitigation of enteric methane emissions in ruminants. Frontiers in Veterinary Science. 2016;**3**:39

[40] Soltan Y, Natel A, Araujo R, Morsy A, Abdalla A. Progressive adaptation of sheep to a microencapsulated blend of essential oils: Ruminal fermentation, methane emission, nutrient digestibility, and microbial protein synthesis. Animal Feed Science and Technology. 2018b;**237**:8-18

[41] Goel G, Makkar HPS. Methane mitigation from ruminants using tannins and saponins, a status review. Tropical Animal Health and Production. 2012;**44**:729-739

[42] Patra AK, Min BR, Saxena J. Dietary tannins on microbial ecology of the gastrointestinal tract in ruminants. In: Patra AK, editor. Dietary Phytochemicals and Microbes. Springer: The Netherlands; 2012. pp. 237-262

[43] Soltan YA, Morsy AS, Sallam SMA, Louvandini H, Abdalla AL. Comparative in vitro evaluation of forage legumes (*Prosopis, Acacia, Atriplex,* and *Leucaena*) on ruminal fermentation and methanogenesis. Journal of Animal and Feed Sciences. 2012;**21**:759-772

[44] Ku-Vera JC, Jiménez-Ocampo R, Valencia-Salazar SS, Montoya-Flores MD, Molina-Botero IC, Arango J, et al. Role of secondary plant metabolites on enteric methane mitigation in ruminants. Frontiers in Veterinary Science. 2020b;**7**:584

[45] Patra AK. Effects of supplementing low-quality roughages with tree foliages on digestibility, nitrogen utilization and rumen characteristics in sheep: a meta-analysis. Journal of Animal Physiology and Animal Nutrition. 2010;**94**:338-353

[46] Pal K, Patra AK, Sahoo A, Kumawat PK. Evaluation of several tropical tree leaves for methane production potential, degradability and rumen fermentation in vitro. Livestock Science. 2015a;**180**:98-105

[47] SoltanYA MAS, Lucas RC, Abdalla AL. Potential of mimosine of *Leucaena leucocephala* for modulating ruminal nutrient degradability and methanogenesis. Animal Feed Science and Technology. 2017;**223**:30-41

[48] Kalinowska M, Zimowski J, Paczkowski C, Wojciechowski ZA. The formation of sugar chains in triterpenoid saponins and glycoalkaloids. Phytochemistry Reviews. 2005;**4**:237-257

[49] Patra AK, Saxena J. The effect and mode of action of saponins on the microbial populations and fermentation in the rumen and ruminant production. Nutrition Research Reviews. 2009;**22**:204-219

[50] Ramos-Morales E, Arco-Pérez A, Martín-García AI, Yáñez-Ruiz DR, Frutos P, Hervás G. Use of stomach tubing as an alternative to rumen cannulation to study ruminal fermentation and microbiota in sheep and goats. Animal Feed Science and Technology. 2014;**198**:57-66

[51] Patra AK. Effects of essential oils on rumen fermentation, microbial ecology and ruminant production. Asian Journal of Animal and Veterinary Advances. 2011;**6**:416-428

[52] Patra AK, Yu Z. Effects of essential oils on methane production and fermentation by, and abundance and diversity of, rumen microbial populations. Applied and Environmental Microbiology. 2012;**78**:4271-4280

[53] Morsy AS, Soltan YA, Sallam SMA, Kreuzer M, Alencar SM, Abdalla AL. Comparison of the in vitro efficiency of supplementary bee propolis extracts of different origin in enhancing the ruminal degradability of organic matter and mitigating the formation of methane. Animal Feed Science and Technology. 2015;**199**:51-60

[54] Soltan YA, Patra AK. Bee propolis as a natural feed additive: bioactive compounds and effects on ruminal fermentation pattern as well as productivity of ruminants. Indian Journal of Animal Health. 2020;**59**:50-61

[55] Morsy AS, Soltan YA, Sallam SM, Alencar SM, Abdalla AL. Impact of Brazilian red propolis extract on blood metabolites, milk production, and lamb performance of Santa Inês ewes. Tropical Animal Health and Production. 2016;**48**:1043-1050

[56] Zhou JH, Li Y, Zhao J, Xue XF, Wu LM, Chen F. Geographical traceability of propolis by high-performance liquid-chromatography fingerprints. Food Chemistry. 2008;**108**:749-759

[57] Costa JBG, Zeoula LM, Franco SL, de Moura LPP, Valero MV, Simioni FL, et al. Effect of propolis product on digestibility and ruminal parameters in buffaloes consuming a forage-based diet. Italian Journal of Animal Science. 2012;**11**:441-448

[58] Morsy AS, Soltan YA, El-Zaiat HM, Alencar SM, Abdalla AL. Role of bee propolis extract on diet digestibility, purine derivatives, mitigating methane formation, and blood metabolites in late pregnant ewes. Animal Feed Science and Technology. 2021;**273**:114834

[59] Patra AK. The effect of dietary fats on methane emissions, and its other effects on digestibility, rumen fermentation and lactation performance in cattle: A meta-analysis. Livestock Science. 2013;**155**:244-254

[60] Wang S, Kreuzer M, Braun U, Schwarm A. Effect of unconventional oilseeds (safflower, poppy, hemp, camelina) on in vitro ruminal methane production and fermentation. Journal of the Science of Food and Agriculture. 2017;**97**:3864-3870

[61] Jiménez-Ocampo R, Valencia-Salazar S, Pinzón-Díaz CE, Herrera-Torres E, Aguilar-Pérez CF, JacoboArango J, et al. The role of chitosan as a possible agent for enteric methane mitigation in ruminants. Animals. 2019;**9**:1-12

[62] Li J, Cai C, Li J, Li J, Li J, SunT WL, et al. Chitosan-based nanomaterials for drug delivery. Molecules. 2018;**23**:2661

[63] Gandra JR, Takiya CS, Oliveira ER, Paiva PG, Goes RHTB, Gandra ÉRS, et al. Nutrient digestion, microbial protein synthesis, and blood metabolites of Jersey heifers fed chitosan and whole raw soybeans. Revista Brasileira de Zootecnia. 2016;**45**:130-137

[64] Zanferari F, Vendramini THA, Rentas MF, Gardinal R, Calomeni GD, Mesquita LG, et al. Effects of chitosan and whole raw soybeans on ruminal fermentation and bacterial populations, and milk fatty acid profile in dairy cows. Journal of Dairy Science. 2018;**101**: 10939-10952

[65] Pal K, Patra AK, Sahoo A, Soren NM. Effects of nitrate and fumarate in tree leaves-based diets on nutrient utilization, rumen fermentation, microbial protein supply and blood profiles in sheep. Livestock Science. 2015b;**172**:5-15

[66] Krause KM, Oetzel GR. Understanding and preventing subacute ruminal acidosis in dairy herds: A review. Animal Feed Science and Technology. 2006;**126**:215-236

[67] Aschenbach JR, Zebeli Q, Patra AK, Greco G, Amasheh S, Penner GB. Symposium review: The importance of the ruminal epithelial barrier for a healthy and productive cow. Journal of Dairy Science. 2019;**102**:1866-1882

[68] Bach A, Guasch I, Elcoso G, Duclos J, Khelil-Arfa H. Modulation of rumen pH by sodium bicarbonate and a blend of different sources of magnesium oxide in lactating dairy cows submitted to a concentrate challenge. Journal of Dairy Science. 2018;**101**:9777-9788

[69] Martin SA, Streeter MN, Nisbet DJ, Hill GM, Williams SE. Effects of DL-malate on ruminal metabolism and performance of cattle fed a high-concentrate diet. Journal of Animal Science. 1999;**77**:1008-1015

[70] Marden JP, Julien C, Monteils V, Auclair E, Moncoulon R, Bayourthe C. How does live yeast differ from sodium bicarbonate to stabilize ruminal pH in high yielding dairy cows? Journal of Dairy Science. 2008;**91**:3528-3535

[71] Razzhi A, Malekkhahi M, Valizadeh R, Parand E, Bayat AR. Modulation of ruminal pH, milk fat secretion, and biohydrogenation intermediates by alkalizing agents in dairy cows fed starch-rich diets. Livestock Science. 2021;**248**:104485

[72] Eckard RJ, Grainger C, De Klein CAM. Options for the abatement of methane and nitrous oxide from ruminant production. Livestock Science. 2010;**130**:47-56

[73] Patra AK. Urea/ammonia metabolism in the rumen and toxicity in ruminants. In: Puniya AK, Singh R, Kamra DN, editors. Rumen Microbiology: From Evolution to Revolution. New Delhi: Springer; 2015. pp. 329-341

[74] Hoover WH, Stokes SR. Balancing carbohydrates and proteins for optimum rumen microbial yield. Journal of Dairy Science. 1991;**74**:3630-3644

[75] Lu Z, Xu Z, Shen Z, Tian Y, Shen H. Dietary energy level promotes rumen microbial protein synthesis by improving the energy productivity of the ruminal microbiome. Frontiers in Microbiology. 2019;**10**:847

[76] Hume ID, Moir RJ, Somers M. Synthesis of microbial protein in the rumen. I. Influence of the level of nitrogen intake. Australian Journal of Agricultural Research. 1970;**21**:283-296

[77] Patra AK, Aschenbach JR. Ureases in the gastrointestinal tracts of ruminant and monogastric animals and their implication in urea-N/ammonia metabolism: A review. Journal of Advanced Research. 2018;**13**:39-50

[78] Patra AK. Exploring the benefits of feeding tannin containing diets for enhancing the nutritional values of milk and meat of ruminants. Indian Journal of Animal Health. 2014;**53**:63-76

[79] Frutosa P, Hervás G, Natalello A, Luciano G, Fondevila M, Priolo A, et al. Ability of tannins to modulate ruminal lipid metabolism and milk and meat fatty acid profiles. Animal Feed Science and Technology. 2020;**269**:114623

[80] Roy A, Mandal GP, Patra AK. Evaluating the performance, carcass traits and conjugated linoleic acid content in muscle and adipose tissues of Black Bengal goats fed soybean oil and sunflower oil. Animal Feed Science and Technology. 2013;**185**:43-52

[81] Vasta V, Luciano G. The effects of dietary consumption of plants secondary compounds on small ruminants' products quality. Small Ruminant Research. 2011;**101**:150-159

Section 3

Environment

Chapter 5

Analysis of Inputs Parameters Used to Estimate Enteric Methane Emission Factors Applying a Tier 2 Model: Case Study of Native Cattle in Senegal

Séga Ndao

Abstract

In the context of the Paris Agreement, and considering the importance of methane emissions from cattle in West Africa, application of a Tier 2 method to estimate enteric methane emission factors is clearly pertinent. The current study has two purposes. Firstly, it aims to detect how much each input parameter contributes to the overall uncertainty of enteric methane emission factors for cattle. Secondly, it aims to identify which input parameters require additional research efforts for strengthening the evidence base, thus reducing the uncertainty of methane enteric emission factors. Uncertainty and sensitivity analysis methodologies were applied to input parameters in the calculation of enteric methane emission factors for lactating cows and adult male Senegalese native cattle using the IPCC Tier 2 model. The results show that the IPCC default input parameters, such as the coefficient for calculating net energy for maintenance (Cf_i), digestible energy (DE) and the methane conversion rate (Y_m) are the first, second and third most important input parameters, respectively, in terms of their contribution to uncertainty of the enteric methane emission factor. Sensitivity analysis demonstrated that future research in Senegal should prioritize the development of Y_m, Cf_i and DE in order to estimate enteric methane emission factors more accurately and to reduce the uncertainty of the national agricultural greenhouse gas inventory.

Keywords: uncertainty analysis, sensitivity analysis, Tier 2 model, native cattle, Senegal

1. Introduction

The important role of the livestock sector in food security is well understood [1]. At the same time, the sector plays a significant role in greenhouse gas emissions to the atmosphere [2, 3]. Among total agriculture sector emissions (5.4 Gt CO2e), 60% is due to livestock emission sources, mostly (63%) enteric fermentation [4].

Within the United Nations Framework Convention on Climate Change (UNFCCC), developing countries are presently required to submit national GHG inventory reports through National Communications. These reports are to be prepared following the Intergovernmental Panel on Climate Change (IPCC) Guidelines for GHG inventories [5]. The 2006 IPCC Guidelines set out three levels (or tiers) of increasing complexity (called Tiers 1–3) for use by a country. The purpose of the tiers is to provide unbiased and accurate estimates of national GHG emissions, and to enable inventory compilers to focus the use of resources on improving accuracy for key emission categories in the inventory. The Tier 1 method provides default values for GHG emissions per head of livestock and can reflect only variation in livestock numbers. The IPCC 2006 Tier 2 method for estimating enteric fermentation emissions from ruminants is based on net energy estimated using the National Research Council model [6]. This approach requires details on the characteristics of livestock sub-categories and their performance, for example, in terms of production (e.g., milk yield, daily weight gain) and reproduction (e.g., percentage of lactating cows).

At present, due to the scarcity of appropriate information on agricultural production in Sub-Saharan Africa (SSA), most countries in this region use the Tier 1 approach to quantify agricultural GHG emissions [7]. However, adopting the IPCC Tier 2 methodology can increase the accuracy of emission estimates [8]. In the SSA region [9, 10], provide enteric methane emission factors (EF) for cattle in South Africa and Benin, respectively, using the Tier 2 approach. A Tier 2 inventory for dairy cattle has also been produced by Kenya [11]. Since its second national communication in 2010, Senegal's national GHG inventory, prepared by the Ministry of Environment, has used EFs calculated using a Tier 2 approach.

However, caution is required when applying the IPCC Tier 2 method to livestock systems in Africa. A recent study reported that the Tier 2 model had low predictive ability when the quality of diet changes [12]. In addition, estimation of enteric methane through the IPCC Tier 2 model assumes that animal is reared in ad libitum conditions throughout the year. In extensive livestock systems such as in West Africa, feedstuffs from grazing resources are typically available in the wet season but is very scarce during the dry season [13–15].

In recent years, further methods have been developed which allow highly accurate determination of emissions [16–18]. However, for developing countries, these measurement techniques may be very expensive and require significant knowledge to implement [19, 20]. Despite its possible shortcomings, therefore, the 2006 IPCC Tier 2 method is a practical method to estimate enteric methane emissions from cattle with greater accuracy than the default Tier 1 method [5].

Implementing a detailed uncertainty and sensitivity analysis of the input parameters in the IPCC Tier 2 model can provide guidance for targeting future research efforts to improve enteric fermentation estimates, with which to inform national GHG inventories, Nationally Appropriate Mitigation Actions (NAMAs) and Nationally Determined Contributions (NDCs).

In this study, the first objective is to use uncertainty analysis (UA) to identify which input parameters contribute significantly to the overall uncertainty of enteric methane emission factors estimated using the IPCC Tier 2 model. The second purpose is to apply sensitivity analysis (SA) in order to identify which parameters, need additional research, thereby increasing the accuracy of enteric methane emission factors.

2. Materials and methods

2.1 Location and livestock grazing systems

Senegal is the most westerly country in Africa with a tropical climate. It covers a surface area of 196,712 square kilometers and has an estimated population of 15.7

million [21]. Approximately 77% of the working population are employed in the agricultural sector [22]. According to the latest population estimates for the year 2018, the rural population represents about 53% of the total population [21]. The estimated ruminant livestock numbers provided by the Senegalese Ministry of Livestock and Animal Production (MEPA) are 3.6 million cattle, 6.7 million sheep and 5.7 million goats [23].

Extensive livestock farming systems in Senegal are based on two native cattle breeds which are found in different agroecological zones. The zebu Gobra (*Bos indicus*) and the taurine Ndama (*Bos taurus*) are mostly raised in the Northern and the Southern parts of Senegal, respectively [24]. The less common Gobra x Ndama crossbreed, termed Djakoré cattle, is located in the Senegalese groundnut basin. To improve national dairy production in Senegal, local cattle breeds are crossed with exotic dairy breeds e.g., Montbelliard, Holstein, through public funded artificial insemination campaigns [25]. To our knowledge, the proportion of the cattle breeds in Senegal has not been officially documented. However, inspection of regional livestock data from MEPA and the distribution area of cattle, our approximations suggest that the zebu Gobra and the taurine Ndama represent 80–90% of the Senegalese cattle population. In this case study, the zebu Gobra and the taurine Ndama cattle, which are the two dominant domestic cattle breeds, are considered. Particularly, lactating cows and adult males are the studied cattle sub-categories.

2.2 Description of the used model

Our evaluation was implemented using the Tier 2 model recommended by IPCC [5]. This model (Eq. (1)) allows to approximate enteric methane emission factors (MEF, kg CH4/head/year) which is the output variable. To calculate gross energy intake (GE, MJ/d), net energy (NE, MJ/d) needed for different metabolic functions (i.e., maintenance, activity, growth, lactation, work and pregnancy) was predicted for each cattle subcategory using various formulas presented in the IPCC Guidelines. The output variable is calculated based on input parameters, such as average live body weight (LW, kg), average daily weight gain (ADG, kg/day), milk production (Milk, kg/day), feeding situation, and digestible energy (DE, %). Finally, these parameters together with the methane (CH4) conversion factor (Ym, %) enable calculation of net energy (NE, MJ/day), average daily feed intake (in terms of gross energy content, MJ/d) and the MEF (i.e., output) for each animal sub-category.

$$EF = \left[\left(GE * \left(Ym / 100\right) * 365\right) / 55.65\right] \tag{1}$$

where:

EF = emission factor, kg CH4 head/yr,

GE = gross energy intake, MJ head/yr,

Ym = methane conversion factor, per cent of gross energy in feed converted to methane.

The factor 55.65, (MJ/kg CH4) is the energy content of methane.

2.3 Sources of input data

The data for input parameters used derived mainly from two Livestock Research Centres (LRC) of the Senegalese Agricultural Research Institute (Institut Sénégalais de Recherches Agricoles, ISRA, see www.isra.sn): the Centre de Recherches

Parameters	Symbol	Unit	References	
			Gobra cattle	Ndama cattle
Coefficient for calculating Net energy for maintenance	Cf_i	MJ/d/kg	[5]	
Activity coefficient corresponding to animal's feed situation	C_a	MJ/d/kg	[5]	
Average live body weight	LW	Kg	CRZ-D database	CRZ-K database
Mature live body weight	MW	Kg	From expert opinion	From expert opinion
Average daily weight gain	ADG	kg/d	[26–28]	CRZ-K Research reports
Coefficient	C	dim.	[5]	
Average daily milk yield	Milk	kg/d	[24]	CRZ-K Research reports
Fat content of milk	Fat	%	[29]	CRZ-K Research reports
Number of hours of work	Hour	H	CRZ-D research reports	CRZ-K research reports
Pregnancy coefficient	C_p	dim.	[5]	
Methane conversion rates	Y_m	%	[5]	
Feed Digestibility	DE	%	[5]	

d: day; dim.: dimensionless; CRZ-D: Centre de Recherches Zootechniques de Dahra; CRZ-K: Centre de Recherches Zootechniques de Kolda.

Table 1.
Input parameters used to estimate enteric methane emission factors for Gobra and Ndama cattle using the Tier 2 methodology and their sources.

Zootechniques de Dahra (CRZ-D) and the Centre de Recherches Zootechniques de Kolda (CRZ-K). These LRCs are located in the Ferlo and the Casamance areas, respectively. The general focus of these LRCs is to disseminate bulls to Senegalese family farms, so as to maintain and improve the productivity (milk and meat) of indigenous cattle. CRZ-D and CRZ-K frequently collect data on reproductive (e.g., rank of calving, calving interval) and productive (e.g., LW, ADG, Milk) performance through surveys and direct measurements implemented as part of research programs conducted independently or in partnership with international research organizations (e.g., CIRAD, FAO).

For this study, research reports, theses, publications and data sourced from ISRA databases (http://intranet.isra.sn/aurifere/opac_css/) were examined for relevant information. Documents (e.g., annual reports) from the Senegalese Livestock Ministry (MEPA, http://www.elevage.gouv.sn/) and the National Agency for Statistics and Demography (ANSD, http://www.ansd.sn) were also consulted. When country-specific data was not available, values from the 2006 IPCC Guidelines for National Greenhouse Gas Inventories was used. **Table 1** presents the data sources used to estimate emission factors for Senegalese cattle breeds.

2.4 Uncertainty and sensitivity analysis procedures

Authors from many scientific fields have described the application of uncertainty analysis (UA) and sensitivity analysis (SA) procedures to various modeling situations [30–32] and for a number of purposes [33]. For example, to achieve comprehensive uncertainty analysis, the 2006 IPCC Guidelines [5] recommend to use the Monte Carlo (MC) simulation method. The MC methodology is useful for dealing with great uncertainties, complex models and existing correlations between parameters [34, 35]. However, expanding the MC domain increases the requirements of the user, in terms of acquiring additional data and designing the analysis, and thus requires strong collaboration between experts [36]. For this present study, analysis of variance (ANOVA) and the standardized regression coefficient (SRC) were implemented for UA and SA, respectively.

Analysis was applied to emission factors for lactating cows (LC) and adult males (MA). The latest national communication indicates that these two animal classes are the largest emission sources among all cattle categories in Senegal [37]. For each of these animal categories, only the relevant parameters were estimated. For example, parameters such as milk yield (Milk, kg/day), fat content of milk (Fat, %) and the coefficient for pregnancy (Cp) were not estimated for MA, while number of hours of work (Hour, h/day) was not estimated for LC. Hence, 11 and 9 input parameters were considered for LC and MA, respectively. The number of simulations were 200,000 and 20,000 for LC and MA, respectively. These numbers were assumed to be satisfactory to stabilize the output. Indeed, a 3-level complete factorial design was defined [38] and considering the K dichotomous input parameters, the design requires 3 K simulations, i.e., 311 and 39 combinations of values for LC and MA, respectively [39].

2.4.1 Uncertainty analysis

Uncertainty analysis (UA) was applied to the enteric methane emission factors (MEF) of Senegalese native cattle derived using the IPCC Tier 2 method.

The input parameters characterized were from two main sources, i.e., parameters with values proposed by the 2006 IPCC Guidelines (PM) and parameters specific to extensive livestock farming systems in Senegal (PS).

The uncertainties of PM expressed in this study were those taken from the literature [5, 40]. The uncertainties of PS were not defined in the Senegalese NIR. Therefore, expert judgment was used to characterize the uncertainty of each PS. To do this, we proceeded as follows. The average value of each PS was estimated using livestock data reported from research conducted in Senegal. Then, these values were shared with national experts for assessment. These national specialists, who had worked previously on countrywide livestock research programs, suggested standard deviations around each mean values of PS, and these were used to represent relative uncertainties of each PS.

Consequently, an uncertainty of ±15% around the value of average live weight (LW, kg) and average daily gain (ADG, kg/day) were assumed. The fitted values of mature weight (MW, kg) had a relative uncertainty of ±25%. Milk production per lactating cow (Milk, kg/day) reported from the extensive livestock farming systems varies widely within and between Senegalese traditional farms, so an uncertainty range of ±20% was assumed, while the value of fat content of milk (Fat, %) was set to randomly fluctuate by ±2%. Regarding feed digestibility (DE, %), an uncertainty of ±15% is most commonly reported in the literature [40–42]. For this study, a value of ±20% was recommended by Senegalese experts, considering the extensive livestock farming systems, which are largely based on the use of rangeland forage resources. The probability density functions (PDFs) of all used input parameters is believed to be symmetrical.

The overall uncertainty in the estimated output is assumed to be normally distributed, with a 95% confidence interval of plus or minus the uncertainty of the assigned value for each input parameter. The **Tables 2** and **3** list the used values of the input parameters, for each breed and animal category.

To estimate the specific contribution of each parameter to overall uncertainty (i.e., uncertainty associated with calculation of enteric methane emission factors), the analysis of variance (ANOVA) procedure was applied. To do this, the uncertainty ranges related to the input parameters were used to define the maximum and minimum values of each input parameter. The distributions were defined as uniform (i.e., normal distributions). Then, using the "runif" instruction, input parameter values were randomly generated using R software [43]. To mimic the contributions of the generated values of each input parameter to output uncertainty, the equations proposed by the IPCC [5] were used. To rank the input parameters according to their effect on the output, the sums of the squares (Sum Sq) computed by the ANOVA procedure for each input parameter were divided by the total sums of squares. Therefore, the results were expressed as a proportion and ordered in terms of percentage contribution to output uncertainty, using the instruction order in the R software. The total uncertainty of enteric methane emission factors was calculated using Rule A [5], which is approximation approach based on first-order Taylor series expansion, often referred to as error propagations [44].

2.4.2 Sensitivity analysis

Some of the SA approach used in this study has been presented previously as a case study (see https://www.agmrv.org) for the Livestock Research Group of the Global Research Alliance for Agricultural Greenhouse Gases (https://globalresearchalliance.org).

A sensitivity package developed by [45] and implemented in R software was used to conduct a global sensitivity analysis procedure [46]. First, to generate values between a minimum and the maximum, we set a range of variation of ±20% around the allocated value of each input parameter, assuming a uniform distribution (with a 95% confidence interval). Second, these values were input into the 2006 IPCC Tier 2 model to generate a range of values for the output. Finally, the standardized

Symbol[1]	Unit	Used value[2]		Uncertainty (±%)	Sources of used uncertainties
		Gobra	Ndama		
ADG	kg/day	0.135	0.110	15	Expert opinion
C	dimensionless	0.8	0.8	30	[40]
C_a	MJ/day/kg	0.36	0.36	30	[40]
Cf_i	MJ/day/kg	0.386	0.386	30	[40]
C_p	dimensionless	0.10	0.10	10	[40]
DE	%	50	50	20	Expert opinion
Fat	%	4.7	4.24	2	Expert opinion
LW	kg	250	200	15	Expert opinion
Milk	kg/day	0.922	0.870	20	Expert opinion
MW	kg	200	180	25	Expert opinion
Y_m	%	6.5	6.5	15	[5]

[1]*For the definition of symbols, see* ***Table 1.***
[2]*For the sources of used values, see* ***Table 1.***

Table 2.
Assigned values of input parameters used in the Tier 2 model to assess enteric methane emission factors for Gobra and Ndama lactating cows.

Symbol[1]	Unit	Used value[2]		Uncertainty (±%)	Sources of used uncertainties
		Gobra	Ndama		
ADG	kg/day	0.135	0.110	15	Expert opinion
C	dimensionless	1.2	1.2	30	[40]
C_a	MJ/day/kg	0.36	0.36	30	[40]
Cf_i	MJ/day/kg	0.37	0.37	30	[40]
DE	%	50	50	20	Expert opinion
Hour	h/day	1.23	1.23	10	Expert opinion
LW	kg	300	250	15	Expert opinion
MW	kg	200	180	25	Expert opinion
Y_m	%	6.5	6.5	15	[5]

[1]*For the definition of symbols, see* ***Table 1.***
[2]*For the sources of used values, see* ***Table 1.***

Table 3.
Assigned values of input parameters used in the Tier 2 model to assess enteric methane emission factors for Gobra and Ndama adult male cattle.

regression coefficient (SRC) was used to obtain sensitivity indices for each input parameter [47]. The SRC reflects the change in the standard deviation of the MEF when all other input parameters are fixed and unchanged [48, 49].

3. Results

3.1 Contribution of input parameters to uncertainty

The estimated values of the effect of each input parameter on overall uncertainty are presented in **Tables 4** and **5** for lactating cows and adult males of the Gobra and Ndama cattle breeds, respectively.

The results show the effect of broad differences in the values for input parameters used in terms of their influence (expressed as a percentage, %) on overall uncertainty. The coefficient for maintenance (Cf_i) contributes more than 55% of the overall uncertainty. Digestibility (DE) and the methane conversion factor (Ym) were the second and third most significant input parameters, respectively. The contributions of the other parameters were less than 10%.

In general, these results were similar for each animal sub-category of each breed, although there was some difference in terms of the contribution of these parameters to overall uncertainty. For example, with respect to lactating cows, the effect of Cf_i on the total uncertainty of the enteric methane EF calculation was greater for Gobra (58.2%) compared to Ndama (54.4%). By comparison, the contribution of Cf_i for adult males was 57.0% and 56.3% for Ndama and Gobra, respectively.

3.2 Sensitivity of used input parameters

Figures 1 and **2** show the standardized regression coefficients (SRC) of each input parameter used to evaluate the enteric methane emission factors for lactating cows and adult males of Senegalese native cattle, respectively.

According to the linear regression method implemented, the methane conversion rate (Y_m) and the coefficient for calculating net energy for maintenance (Cf_i) are the parameters with the largest SRC. The results show also the importance of the digestibility of feed (DE%) and liveweight (LW). The rank order in terms

Species	Parameters	Sum sq	Mean sq	F value	Pr (>F)	Contribution (%)
Gobra	Cf_i	6302301	6302301	7319021	0.000	58.2
	DE	2064336	2064336	2397366	0.000	19.1
	Y_m	1823864	1823864	2118099	0.000	16.8
	C_a	350673	350673	407245	0.000	3.2
	LW	96244	96244	111770	0.000	0.9
	Milk	20210	20210	23470	0.000	0.2
	C_p	3330	3330	3867	0.000	0.0
	ADG	109	109	127	0.000	0.0
	Fat	83	83	96	0.000	0.0
	C	66	66	77	0.000	0.0
	MW	16	16	18	0.000	0.0
	Residuals	172207	1	NA	NA	1.6
Ndama	Cf_i	4509591	4509591	6005876	0.000	54.4
	DE	1438224	1438224	1915428	0.000	17.3
	Y_m	1293936	1293936	1723265	0.000	15.6
	LW	625802	625802	833444	0.000	7.5
	C_a	253737	253737	337927	0.000	3.1
	Milk	15579	15579	20748	0.000	0.2
	C_p	2938	2938	3913	0.000	0.0
	Fat	119	119	158	0.000	0.0
	MW	72	72	95	0.000	0.0
	C	68	68	90	0.000	0.0
	ADG	0	0	0	0.659	0.0
	Residuals	150164	1	NA	NA	1.8

NA: not applicable.

Table 4.
Contribution to the overall uncertainty of input parameters used to calculate enteric methane emission factors for lactating cows of Senegalese native cattle breeds.

Species	Parameters	Sum sq	Mean sq	F value	Pr (>F)	Contribution (%)
Gobra	Cf_i	760631	760631	605099	0.000	56.3
	DE	216733	216733	172416	0.000	16.0
	Y_m	195408	195408	155451	0.000	14.5
	LW	107049	107049	85160	0.000	7.9
	C_a	46181	46181	36738	0.000	3.4
	Hour	646	646	514	0.000	0.0
	ADG	8	8	6	0.014	0.0
	C	2	2	1	0.241	0.0
	MW	0	0	0	0.536	0.0
	Residuals	25128	1	NA	NA	1.9

Species	Parameters	Sum sq	Mean sq	F value	Pr (>F)	Contribution (%)
Ndama	Cf_i	595693	595693	611755	0.000	57.0
	DE	161026	161026	165368	0.000	15.4
	Y_m	148597	148597	152604	0.000	14.2
	LW	82999	82999	85237	0.000	7.9
	C_a	37722	37722	38739	0.000	3.6
	Hour	276	276	284	0.000	0.0
	MW	14	14	15	0.000	0.0
	C	1	1	1	0.273	0.0
	ADG	0	0	0	0.746	0.0
	Residuals	19465	1	NA	NA	1.9

NA: not applicable.

Table 5.
Contribution to the overall uncertainty of input parameters used to calculate enteric methane emission factors for adult male Senegalese native cattle breeds.

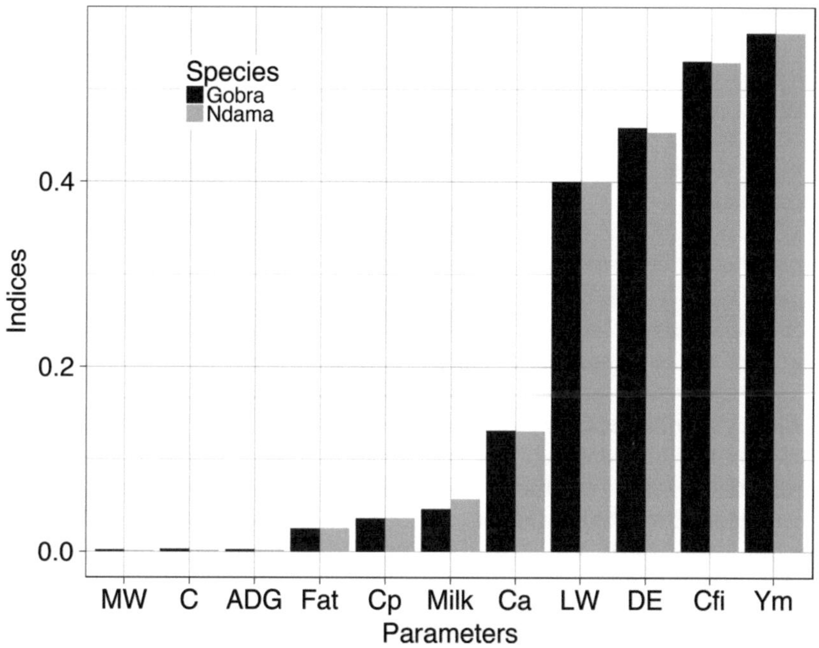

Figure 1.
Sensitivity indices based on standardized regression coefficients of input parameters used to calculate enteric methane emission factors for lactating cows of Senegalese native cattle breeds.

of sensitivity was identical for both cattle breeds and each animal sub-category. Moreover, our results reveal that among breeds, the SRC obtained for Ndama cattle was slightly larger. Differences were also observed between sub-categories. Compared to lactating cows, the SRC was higher for adult male Gobra cattle for parameters such as Y_m, Cf_i, and LW. For lactating cows, compared with adult males, Ym and DE showed more sensitivity for Ndama cattle. However, irrespective of breed or sub-category, the differences observed between SRC of input parameters did not exceed 8%.

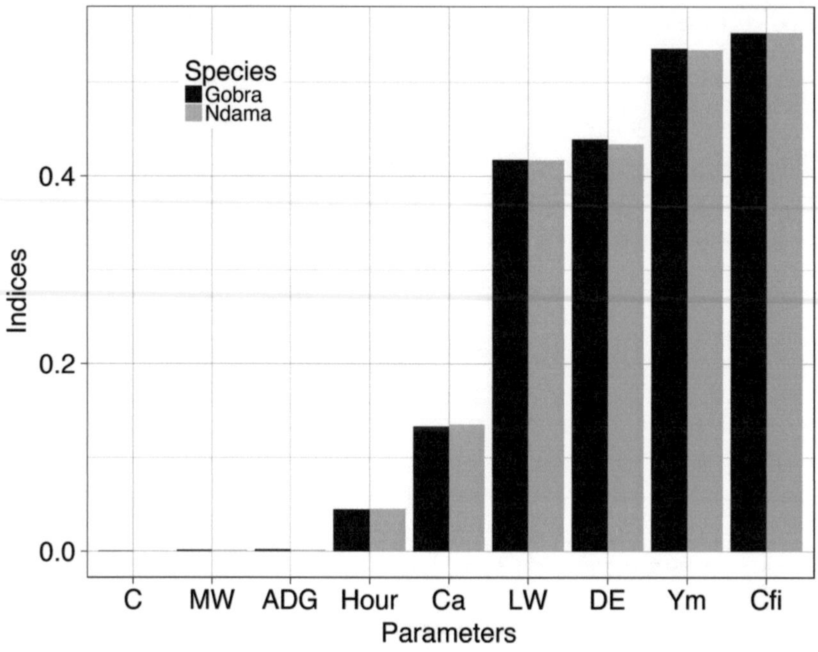

Figure 2.
Sensitivity indices based on standardized regression coefficients of input parameters used to calculate enteric methane emission factors for adult males of Senegalese native cattle breeds.

4. Discussion

4.1 Moving to a Tier 2 enteric methane emission factor

To date, because of the scarcity of relevant data in developing countries in the SSA region, the Tier 1 approach is most commonly used to evaluate enteric methane emission from livestock [50, 51]. Assessments at the regional level suggest that Africa has a higher uncertainty for each livestock product compared with Europe [52]. Additionally, [8] reported that only about one third of countries located in developing regions have conducted evaluation of uncertainty in their national GHG inventory. Considering the absence of reliable information on livestock in the SSA region, the IPCC Guidelines suggest that the uncertainty of enteric fermentation emission factors ranges from ±30% to ±50% for Tier 1 and ± 20% for Tier 2 approaches, respectively [5]. Hence, the use of a Tier 2 approach may enable a decrease in the uncertainty of predicted enteric methane emission factors used in national GHG inventories [53–55]. In Senegal, the third GHG emission inventory was submitted to the UNFCCC in 2015 (see https://unfccc.int/documents/89618). In that inventory, enteric methane emission of cattle was assessed using the Tier 2 methodology. Within the overall emissions from the agricultural sector, enteric methane was identified as a key source of emissions (accounting for 72% of total agricultural emissions). Cattle were responsible for 65% of total agricultural emissions. However, uncertainty analysis has not previously been performed on that national GHG inventory.

4.2 Importance of input parameters

Considering the results of both uncertainty and sensitivity analysis computed in this study, our calculations indicate that the coefficient of maintenance (Cf_i), the digestibility of feed (DE) and the methane conversion factor (Y_m) are the input parameters which require further research, because of their influence on the accuracy of enteric methane emission factors calculated using the 2006 IPCC Tier 2 approach.

The importance of Cf_i has been pointed out in previous research conducted in other regions [41, 42, 53]. The value of Cfi implemented in our assessment was sourced from the IPCC Guidelines. To our knowledge, studies focusing on this parameter are very few, particularly in developing countries, despite the dependence of this parameter on variation in temperature [5].

The composition of fodder consumed by ruminants is well documented in Senegal, and the profile of organic matter digestibility (OMd) is available [13–15, 54]. However, there is a need to determine at the national scale, an average value for OMd which takes into consideration seasonality. To date, the default value for feed digestibility (DE, %) from the IPCC Guidelines (i.e., 50 ± 5%) has always been applied in the Senegalese national GHG inventory. In general, estimation of DE is very complex, considering the various factors which need to be taken into consideration [56–58]. To estimate DE, robust formula needs to be developed based on numerous data which consider the diversity of diet [59]. For example, in West African livestock farming systems, the largest proportion of feed is from natural pastures [60–62]. Cattle herds in this region graze different types of feedstuffs (e.g., trees, crop residues, woody species, grasses). Throughout the seasons, the composition of the diet and the nutrient content of feedstuff both fluctuate [13, 63, 64]. Given the diversity of feedstuff and seasonal fluctuations in the West African context, determining an annual average value of DE is challenging. A fixed value for DE is reasonable as it is supposed to represent the annual average. Additionally, apart from the proposed values of DE in the 2006 IPCC Guidelines, reports of the value of DE are very limited in the literature, even in some developed countries. Indeed, with the lack of country-specific data related to the feeding system, Belgium applies DE values from the Netherlands, assuming that feed systems are comparable [65]. Slovenia uses a predicted equation sourced from INRA and German feeding tables [66]. In the national inventory of the UK, the DE values applied for dairy cattle were from tables of nutritive value and chemical composition of feeds, while for beef cattle values were based on expert opinion [67].

The methane conversion factor (Y_m, %) is the third parameter which needs to be better estimated when using the Tier 2 approach. Ym is defined as the percent of gross energy intake that is converted into methane (kg CH4/kg GEI). The appropriate value of Ym is the subject of considerable research by scientists [68]. Using a meta-analysis approach, [69] propose using 8.4 ± 0.4% (range 4.8% to 13.7%) for Y_m, while [70] suggest a value which varies from 5.0% to 7.2%. Several countries apply values for Y_m other than the default values suggested by the 2006 IPCC Guidelines. For example, Croatia calculated Y_m using a model reported by [56]. Denmark used a value for Y_m for dairy cattle (ranging from 5.98% to 6.13%) reported by [71].

Hence, in view of the diverse diet composition consumed by cattle over the course of the seasons in West Africa [72–74], determination of an appropriate value for Ym is clearly important for estimating the expected enteric methane emission factor using the IPCC 2006 Tier 2 approach.

In our case, we used expert judgment to characterize the uncertainties of input parameters. In addition, it is possible that the inputs parameters can be correlated. In Senegal, due to the scarcity of relevant reports related to the percentage of native cattle breeds in the total cattle herd, it is probable that uncertainty of activity data is actually higher than uncertainty of emission factors and should be a priority for GHG inventory improvement.

5. Conclusions

The purpose of conducting uncertainty and sensitivity analysis was to identify the most important factors driving emission factors in order to prioritize future data improvement and research efforts so as to improve livestock GHG emission estimates and reduce the uncertainty of inventory estimates for Senegal. Having applied analysis of variance and regression techniques for uncertainty analysis and sensitivity analysis, respectively, our results suggest that future research should focus on the estimates of the coefficient of maintenance, feed digestibility and the methane conversion factor.

Acknowledgements

We thank colleagues who contributed to improving this manuscript.

Conflict of interest

The author declares that no conflicts of interest have affected the conduct of the work proposed in this paper.

Author details

Séga Ndao
ISRA, Centre de Recherches Zootechniques de Kolda, Kolda, Senegal

*Address all correspondence to: ndaosega@gmail.com

References

[1] Godber, O. F., & Wall, R. (2014). Livestock and food security: vulnerability to population growth and climate change. Global change biology, 20(10), 3092-3102.

[2] Steinfeld, H., Gerber, P., Wassenaar, T. D., Castel, V., Rosales, M., Rosales, M., & de Haan, C. (2006). Livestock's long shadow: environmental issues and options. Food & Agriculture Org.

[3] Gerber, P. J., Steinfeld, H., Henderson, B., Mottet, A., Opio, C., Dijkman, J., ... & Tempio, G. (2013). Tackling climate change through livestock: a global assessment of emissions and mitigation opportunities. Food and Agriculture Organization of the United Nations (FAO).

[4] Tubiello, F. N., Cóndor-Golec, R. D., Salvatore, M., Piersante, A., Federici, S., Ferrara, A., ... & Jacobs, H. (2015). Estimating greenhouse gas emissions in agriculture: a manual to address data requirements for developing countries. Estimating greenhouse gas emissions in agriculture: a manual to address data requirements for developing countries.

[5] Eggleston, S., Buendia, L., Miwa, K., Ngara, T., & Tanabe, K. (Eds.). (2006). 2006 IPCC guidelines for national greenhouse gas inventories (Vol. 5). Hayama, Japan: Institute for Global Environmental Strategies.

[6] National Research Council. (1989). Recommended dietary allowances. National Academies Press.

[7] Rosenstock, T. S., Rufino, M. C., Butterbach-Bahl, K., & Wollenberg, E. (2013). Toward a protocol for quantifying the greenhouse gas balance and identifying mitigation options in smallholder farming systems. Environmental Research Letters, 8(2), 021003.

[8] Wilkes, A., Reisinger, A., Wollenberg, E. and van Dijk, S. (2017). Measurement, reporting and verification of livestock GHG emissions by developing countries in the UNFCCC: current practices and opportunities for improvement. CCAFS Report No. 17. CGIAR Research Program on Climate Change, Agriculture and Food Security (CCAFS) and Global Research Alliance for Agricultural Greenhouse Gases (GRA).

[9] Du Toit, C. J. L., Meissner, H. H., & Van Niekerk, W. A. (2013). Direct methane and nitrous oxide emissions of South African dairy and beef cattle. South African Journal of Animal Science, 43(3), 320-339.

[10] Kouazounde, J. B., Gbenou, J. D., Babatounde, S., Srivastava, N., Eggleston, S. H., Antwi, C., ... & McAllister, T. A. (2015). Development of methane emission factors for enteric fermentation in cattle from Benin using IPCC Tier 2 methodology. animal, 9(3), 526-533.

[11] State Department for Livestock (SDL). (2020). Inventory of GHG emissions from dairy cattle in Kenya 1994-2017. State Department for Livestock, Nairobi. http://www.kilimo.go.ke/wp-content/uploads/2020/07/Kenya-Dairy-Cattle-GHG-inventory-Report_06_07_2020.pdf

[12] Benaouda, M., Martin, C., Li, X., Kebreab, E., Hristov, A. N., Yu, Z., ... & Bannink, A. (2019). Evaluation of the performance of existing mathematical models predicting enteric methane emissions from ruminants: animal categories and dietary mitigation strategies. Animal Feed Science and Technology, 114207.

[13] Ickowicz, A., and Mbaye, M. (2001). Forêts soudaniennes et alimentation des bovins au Sénégal:

potentiel et limites. Bois et forêts des tropiques, (270), 47-61.

[14] Chirat, G., Groot, J. C., Messad, S., Bocquier, F., & Ickowicz, A. (2014). Instantaneous intake rate of free-grazing cattle as affected by herbage characteristics in heterogeneous tropical agro-pastoral landscapes. Applied Animal Behaviour Science, 157, 48-60.

[15] Assouma, M. H., Lecomte, P., Hiernaux, P., Ickowicz, A., Corniaux, C., Decruyenaere, V., ... & Vayssières, J. (2018). How to better account for livestock diversity and fodder seasonality in assessing the fodder intake of livestock grazing semi-arid sub-Saharan Africa rangelands. Livestock Science, 216, 16-23.

[16] Kebreab, E., Johnson, K. A., Archibeque, S. L., Pape, D., & Wirth, T. (2008). Model for estimating enteric methane emissions from United States dairy and feedlot cattle. Journal of animal science, 86(10), 2738-2748.

[17] Goopy, J. P., Woodgate, R., Donaldson, A., Robinson, D. L., & Hegarty, R. S. (2011). Validation of a short-term methane measurement using portable static chambers to estimate daily methane production in sheep. Animal Feed Science and Technology, 166, 219-226.

[18] Huhtanen, P., Ramin, M., & Hristov, A. N. (2019). Enteric methane emission can be reliably measured by the GreenFeed monitoring unit. Livestock science, 222, 31-40.

[19] Powers, W., Auvermann, B., Cole, A., Gooch, C., Grant, R., Hatfield, J., . . . Powell, J. M. (2014). Chapter 5: Quantifying Greenhouse Gas Sources and Sinks in Animal Production Systems. In Quantifying Greenhouse Gas Fluxes in Agriculture and Forestry: Methods for Entity-Scale Inventory. Office of the Chief Economist, U.S. Department of Agriculture. Washington. DC.: USDA

[20] Hammond, K. J., Crompton, L. A., Bannink, A., Dijkstra, J., Yáñez-Ruiz, D. R., O'Kiely, P., ... & Schwarm, A. (2016). Review of current in vivo measurement techniques for quantifying enteric methane emission from ruminants. Animal Feed Science and Technology, 219, 13-30.

[21] ANSD. (2018). Rapport projection de la population du Sénégal en 2018. Division du recensement et des statistiques démographiques. Direction des statisques démongraphiques et sociales. Accessed August 10, 2019: http://www.ansd.sn/ressources/publications/Rapport_population_060219%20002%20RECsn%20.pdf.

[22] Roy-Macauley, H., Zougmoré, R., Nelson, G. C., & Jalloh, A. (2017). L'agriculture Ouest-Africaine et le changement climatique. Intl Food Policy Res Inst.

[23] MEPA. (2016). Rapport d'activités du Ministère de l'Elevage et des Productions Animales. Available at : http://www.elevage.gouv.sn/sites/default/files/Rapport_MEPA_2016.pdf

[24] ISRA. (2005). Bilan de la recherche agricole et agroalimentaire au Sénégal. Institut Sénégalais de Recherches Agricoles. Dakar. ISRA-ITA-CIRAD.

[25] Marshall, K., Gibson, J. P., Mwai, O., Mwacharo, J. M., Haile, A., Getachew, T., ... & Kemp, S. J. (2019). Livestock Genomics for Developing Countries–African Examples in Practice. Frontiers in genetics, 10.

[26] Sow, I., S. R., Denis, J., Trail, J., Thiongane, P., Mbaye, M., & Diallo. 1988. (1988). Productivité du zébu Gobra au Centre de Recherches Zootechniques de Dahra (Senegal). Institut Sénégalais de Recherches

Agricoles, Recherches Sante et Productions Animales. Unival.

[27] Diop, M. (1990). Les Systèmes d'élevage Dans Le Ferlo : Etude synthétique de la Situation actuelle. Papier préparé pour le séminaire sur "Les systèmes de production de lait et de viande au Sahel. ISRA-EISMV.

[28] Mbaye, M., Diop, M. and Ndiaye, M. (1991). Etude de la puberté et des paramètres de production du zebu Gobra en milieu traditionnel. ISRA-EISMV.

[29] Kalandi, M., Sow, A., Guigma, W. V. H., Zabre, M. Z., Bathily, A., & Sawadogo, G. J. (2015). Evaluation de la qualité nutritionnelle du lait cru dans les élevages traditionnels de Kaolackau Sénégal. International Journal of Biological and Chemical Sciences, 9(2), 901-909.

[30] Saltelli, Andrea. (2002). Sensitivity analysis for importance assessment. Risk Analysis 22 (3): 579-590.

[31] Makowski, D., Naud, C., Jeuffroy, M. H., Barbottin, A., & Monod, H. (2006). Global sensitivity analysis for calculating the contribution of genetic parameters to the variance of crop model prediction. Reliability Engineering & System Safety, 91(10-11), 1142-1147.

[32] Iooss, B. (2011). Revue sur l'analyse de sensibilité globale de modèles numériques. Journal de la Société Française de Statistique, 152(1), 1-23.

[33] Hamby, D. M. (1994). A review of techniques for parameter sensitivity analysis of environmental models. Environmental monitoring and assessment, 32(2), 135-154.

[34] Gibbons, J. M., Ramsden, S. J., & Blake, A. (2006). Modelling uncertainty in greenhouse gas emissions from UK agriculture at the farm level. Agriculture, ecosystems & environment, 112(4), 347-355.

[35] Ortiz-Gonzalo, D., Vaast, P., Oelofse, M., de Neergaard, A., Albrecht, A., & Rosenstock, T. S. (2017). Farm-scale greenhouse gas balances, hotspots and uncertainties in smallholder crop-livestock systems in Central Kenya. Agriculture, Ecosystems & Environment, 248, 58-70.

[36] Fauser, P., Sørensen, P. B., Nielsen, M., Winther, M., Plejdrup, M. S., Hoffmann, L., ... & Thomsen, M. (2011). Monte Carlo (Tier 2) uncertainty analysis of Danish Greenhouse gas emission inventory. Greenhouse Gas Measurement and Management, 1(3-4), 145-160.

[37] Senegal NIR. (2015). Accessed June 6, 2019 at: https://unfccc.int/sites/default/files/resource/Sennc3.pdf.

[38] Makowski, D. (2013). Objectifs et principales étapes de l'analyse d'incertitude et de sensibilité. Analyse de sensibilité et exploration de modèles. Editions Quae, Versailles, 3-30.

[39] Dziak, J. J., Nahum-Shani, I., & Collins, L. M. (2012). Multilevel factorial experiments for developing behavioral interventions: Power, sample size, and resource considerations. Psychological methods, 17(2), 153.

[40] Monni, S., Perälä, P., & Regina, K. (2007). Uncertainty in agricultural CH 4 and N 2 O emissions from Finland–possibilities to increase accuracy in emission estimates. Mitigation and adaptation strategies for global change, 12(4), 545-571.

[41] Karimi-Zindashty, Y., MacDonald, J. D., Desjardins, R. L., Worth, D. E., Hutchinson, J. J., & Vergé, X. P. C. (2012). Sources of uncertainty in the IPCC Tier 2 Canadian livestock model. The Journal of Agricultural Science, 150(5), 556-569.

[42] Milne, A. E., Glendining, M. J., Bellamy, P., Misselbrook, T., Gilhespy, S., Casado, M. R., ... & Whitmore, A. P. (2014). Analysis of uncertainties in the estimates of nitrous oxide and methane emissions in the UK's greenhouse gas inventory for agriculture. Atmospheric Environment, 82, 94-105.

[43] Team, R. C. (2020). R: A language and environment for statistical computing. R Foundation for Statistical Computing, Vienna, Austria. Retrieved December 24, 2018, from https://www.r-project.org.

[44] Wu, S. J., & Hsu, C. T. (2018). Modeling of uncertainty for flood wave propagation induced by variations in initial and boundary conditions using expectation operator on explicit numerical solutions. International Journal for Numerical Methods in Engineering, 113(9), 1447-1465.

[45] Pujol, G., Iooss, B., Janon, A., Gilquin, L., Le Gratiet, L. and Lemaitre, P. (2012). Package `sensitivity': Sensitivity Analysis. R Package Version 1.5.

[46] Saltelli, A., Ratto, M., Andres, T., Campolongo, F., Cariboni, J., Gatelli, D., ... & Tarantola, S. (2008). Global sensitivity analysis: the primer. John Wiley & Sons.

[47] Saltelli, A., Tarantola, S., & Chan, K. S. (1999). A quantitative model-independent method for global sensitivity analysis of model output. Technometrics, 41(1), 39-56.

[48] Lee Rodgers, J., & Nicewander, W. A. (1988). Thirteen ways to look at the correlation coefficient. The American Statistician, 42(1), 59-66.

[49] Saporta, G. (2006). Probabilités, analyse des données et statistique. Editions Technip.

[50] Ma, L., Zhong, M., Zhu, Y., Yang, H., Johnson, D. A., & Rong, Y. (2018). Annual methane budgets of sheep grazing systems were regulated by grazing intensities in the temperate continental steppe: A two-year case study. Atmospheric environment, 174, 66-75.

[51] Ndung'u, P. W., Bebe, B. O., Ondiek, J. O., Butterbach-Bahl, K., Merbold, L., & Goopy, J. P. (2019). Improved region-specific emission factors for enteric methane emissions from cattle in smallholder mixed crop: livestock systems of Nandi County, Kenya. Animal Production Science, 59(6), 1136-1146.

[52] Zhu, B., Kros, J., Lesschen, J. P., Staritsky, I. G., & de Vries, W. (2016). Assessment of uncertainties in greenhouse gas emission profiles of livestock sectors in Africa, Latin America and Europe. Regional Environmental Change, 16(6), 1571-1582.

[53] Patra, A. K. (2012). Estimation of methane and nitrous oxide emissions from Indian livestock. Journal of Environmental Monitoring, 14(10), 2673-2684.

[54] Doreau, M., Benhissi, H., Thior, Y. E., Bois, B., Leydet, C., Genestoux, L., ... & Ickowicz, A. (2016). Methanogenic potential of forages consumed throughout the year by cattle in a Sahelian pastoral area. Animal Production Science, 56(3), 613-618.

[55] Hristov, A. N., Kebreab, E., Niu, M., Oh, J., Bannink, A., Bayat, A. R., ... & Dijkstra, J. (2018). Symposium review: Uncertainties in enteric methane inventories, measurement techniques, and prediction models. Journal of dairy science, 101(7), 6655-6674.

[56] Hristov, A. N., Oh, J., Firkins, J. L., Dijkstra, J., Kebreab, E., Waghorn, G., ... & Gerber, P. J. (2013). Special topics—Mitigation of methane and nitrous oxide emissions from animal operations: I. A

review of enteric methane mitigation options. Journal of animal science, 91(11), 5045-5069.

[57] Descheemaeker, K., Oosting, S. J., Tui, S. H. K., Masikati, P., Falconnier, G. N., & Giller, K. E. (2016). Climate change adaptation and mitigation in smallholder crop–livestock systems in sub-Saharan Africa: a call for integrated impact assessments. Regional Environmental Change, 16(8), 2331-2343.

[58] Brandt, P., Herold, M., & Rufino, M. C. (2018). The contribution of sectoral climate change mitigation options to national targets: a quantitative assessment of dairy production in Kenya. Environmental Research Letters, 13(3), 034016.

[59] Eugène, M., Sauvant, D., Nozière, P., Viallard, D., Oueslati, K., Lherm, M., ... & Doreau, M. (2019). A new Tier 3 method to calculate methane emission inventory for ruminants. Journal of environmental management, 231, 982-988.

[60] Gautier, D., Bonnérat, A., & Njoya, A. (2005). The relationship between herders and trees in space and time in northern Cameroon. Geographical Journal, 171(4), 324-339.

[61] Ouédraogo-Koné, S., Kaboré-Zoungrana, C. Y., & Ledin, I. (2006). Behaviour of goats, sheep and cattle on natural pasture in the sub-humid zone of West Africa. Livestock Science, 105(1-3), 244-252.

[62] Tongwane, M. I., & Moeletsi, M. E. (2018). A review of greenhouse gas emissions from the agriculture sector in Africa. Agricultural Systems, 166, 124-134.

[63] Touré, S. F., Michalet-Doreau, B., Traoré, E., Friot, D., & Richard, D. (1998). Occurrence of digestive interactions in tree forage-based diets for sheep. Animal Feed Science and Technology, 74(1), 63-78.

[64] Amole T.A., Ayantunde A. A. (2016). Climate-smart livestock interventions in West Africa: A review. CCAFS Working Paper no. 178. CGIAR Research Program on Climate Change, Agriculture and Food Security (CCAFS). Copenhagen, Denmark: CGIAR Research Program on Climate Change, Agriculture and Food Security (CCAFS).

[65] Belgium NIR (2018). Accessed August 20, 2019 at: https://unfccc.int/documents/65711

[66] Slovenia NIR. (2018). Accessed June 6, 2019 at: https://unfccc.int/documents/65714

[67] UK NIR. (2018). Accessed August 22, 2019 at: https://unfccc.int/documents/65762

[68] Van Lingen, H. J., Niu, M., Kebreab, E., Valadares Filho, S. C., Rooke, J. A., Duthie, C. A., ... & Eugène, M. (2019). Prediction of enteric methane production, yield and intensity of beef cattle using an intercontinental database. Agriculture, Ecosystems & Environment, 283, 106575.

[69] Kaewpila, C., & Sommart, K. (2016). Development of methane conversion factor models for Zebu beef cattle fed low-quality crop residues and by-products in tropical regions. Ecology and evolution, 6(20), 7422-7432.

[70] Kennedy, P. M., & Charmley, E. (2012). Methane yields from Brahman cattle fed tropical grasses and legumes. Animal Production Science, 52(4), 225-239.

[71] Hellwing, A. L. F., Weisbjerg, M. R., Brask, M., Alstrup, L., Johansen, M., Hymøller, L., ... & Lund, P. (2016). Prediction of the methane conversion factor (Ym) for dairy cows on the basis

of national farm data. Animal production science, 56(3), 535-540.

[72] Archimède, H., Eugène, M., Magdeleine, C. M., Boval, M., Martin, C., Morgavi, D. P., ... & Doreau, M. (2011). Comparison of methane production between C3 and C4 grasses and legumes. Animal Feed Science and Technology, 166, 59-64.

[73] Nicholson, S. E. (2013). The West African Sahel: A review of recent studies on the rainfall regime and its interannual variability. ISRN Meteorology, 2013.

[74] Taugourdeau, S., Daget, P., Chatelain, C., Mathieu, D., Juanes, X., Huguenin, J., & Ickowicz, A. (2019). FLOTROP, a massive contribution to plant diversity data for open ecosystems in northern tropical africa. Scientific data, 6(1), 118.

Chapter 6

Effect of Various Feed Additives on the Methane Emissions from Beef Cattle Based on an Ammoniated Palm Frond Feeds

Mardiati Zain, Rusmana Wijaya Setia Ningrat, Heni Suryani and Novirman Jamarun

Abstract

Methane gas has a very significant contribution to the increase in greenhouse gases (GHG) globally. The livestock sector, especially ruminants, causes the issue of increasing GHG concentrations. The chapter presents the issue of reducing methane gas production from cattle. Various experiments to reduce methane gas production from ruminants have been carried out and have shown varying results. This series of results of the author's research on reducing methane gas production in livestock in beef cattle based on agriculture by-product to animal feed is addressed with this background. Agriculture by-products such as oil palm fronds and rice straw can be used to feed beef cattle in Indonesia. However, agriculture by-product as animal feed can reduce feed efficiency and increase methane gas production due to the high lignin content. Therefore, various alternatives are carried out to optimize the utilization of this plantation waste. One of them is the use of feed additives and methanogenesis inhibitors. The author's series of research using feed additives (direct-fed microbial) and various methanogenesis inhibitors (plant bioactive compounds and dietary lipids) were tested to determine their effect on nutrient digestibility and methane gas production in feed based on plantation waste. Experiments were carried out *in vitro* and *in vivo* on various types of ruminants. Plant bioactive compounds such as tannins are proven to reduce methane production through their ability to defaunate in the rumen. Tannins may also have direct effect on methanogens and indirectly by reducing fiber digestion. In addition, direct-fed microbial (DFM) feed additives such as *Saccharomyces cerevisiae, Bacillus amyloliquifaciens, and Aspergillus oryz*ae can be used in ruminants to increase livestock productivity. Furthermore, virgin coconut oil as a dietary lipid contains medium-chain fatty acids, mainly lauric acid, which can inhibit the development of ciliates of protozoa and methanogenic bacteria that produce methane in the rumen.

Keywords: feed additive, direct fed microbials, virgin coconut oils, tannins and saponin, methane emissions, beef cattle, ammoniated palm frond

1. Introduction

The main problem in the development of ruminant livestock production in Indonesia, such as beef cattle, is the difficulty of meeting the availability of forage sustainably, both in quality and quantity. Therefore, the use of plantation waste such as palm fronds, rice straw as animal feed is an alternative that can be done to overcome the problem of feed availability. The utilization of plantation waste as ruminant feed is still minimal due to the high content of lignin [1] which causes low digestibility [1–3]. To optimize plantation waste as animal feed, it is necessary to combine processing techniques and optimize bioprocesses in the rumen [3], which aims to increase the microbial population and streamline the fermentation process in the rumen.

Supplementation of direct-fed microbial (DFM) and methanogenesis inhibitors is a way that can be done to increase the efficiency of rumen fermentation [3–5]. DFM is a feed additive product that contains a source of live microorganisms [6], can modify the rumen ecosystem [7], synthesize nutrients so that their availability can increase livestock growth [8]. *S. cerevisiae* is one of the DFM microbes that can be added together with other bacteria and fungi such as Aspergillus sp. and Bacillus sp. [3]. The administration of S. cerevisiae as an additive to live microbes into the body will affect the host by improving the balance of rumen microorganisms [9]. *S. cerevisiae* can compete with starch bacteria [10].

High-fiber feeds such as plantation waste reduce not only the efficiency of feed use [11] but also increase the production of methane gas (CH4) [12]. In the livestock sector, methane is one of the gaseous products of fermented feed ingredients by rumen microbes. Ruminants account for more than 75% of methane emissions from total greenhouse emissions [13]. The release of methane causes an increase in the concentration of CH4 in the air and causes energy loss of 6–13% from the feed [14]. Many livestock nutritionists try to reduce methane production because they feel responsible for the contribution of the livestock sector to atmospheric pollution by methane, as one of the pollutants that is always associated with global warming [15]. Decreased methane production in the rumen is closely related to the metabolic activity of protozoa [16]. Ciliated protozoa in the rumen are in symbiosis with methane bacteria, so that by reducing the population of ciliated protozoa, it will reduce the availability of hydrogen for the formation of methane [17].

Tannins are plant bioactive compounds that can reduce methane production because they act as protozoal defaunation agents [18]. The results of the meta-analysis of *in vivo* experiments with tannins reported by Jayanegara et al., [19] revealed that the concentration of tannins is closely related to the production of CH4 produced. Different sources of tannins have been shown to have different impacts on CH4 production. This is probably because the composition and types of tannins [12] are different from different sources. In addition to tannins, Virgin coconut oil (VCO) contains many medium-chain fatty acids (MCFA). Medium-chain fatty acids (MCFA) are known to have a high potential to suppress rumen methanogenic bacteria [20]. The most abundant MCFA in VCO was lauric acid (C12: 0) 51.95% [21]. Soliva *et al.*, [22] stated that lauric acid (C12: 0) is more effective in suppressing methanogenesis than myristic acid (C14: 0). The ability of VCO to modify the rumen ecosystem depends on the level of its addition in the feed [23]. The high lauric acid content in VCO will allow VCO to have the ability as a defaunation agent against ciliated protozoa and inhibit archaea methanogens in the rumen.

Based on the description above, this chapter book presents several reviews of the results of the author's research, which combines a combination of processing techniques and optimization of bioprocesses in the rumen to increase the value of benefits from plantation waste that can be packaged into complete quality rations, able to increase livestock productivity and reduce beef cattle methane production.

2. Direct fed microbial and virgin coconut oils on methane gas production

2.1 Effect direct-fed microbes on rumen microbial population

Direct-fed microbes (DFM) have comparable results to probiotics. DFM is a feed product that contains a source of live microorganisms [6]. DFM is commonly used as a supplement to increase livestock production. DFM commonly used in ruminants is yeast. DFM works to modify the rumen ecosystem to create an optimal environment for the development of rumen microbes. The provision of DFM as an additive to live microbes in the feed will affect the host by improving the balance of rumen microorganisms [9].

The three-stage series of research has been conducted by Suryani *et al.*, [3]. Phase I is a research aimed at optimizing the bioprocess in the rumen through DFM to increase the rumen microbial population. Three types of DFM were used, namely *Saccharomyces cerevisiae*, *Aspergillus oryzae*, and *Bacillus amyloliquefacien*. The substrate used was based on palm frond, which had previously been ammoniated using 6% urea. The evaluation was carried out *in vitro* [24] to determine nutrient degradation and rumen fermentability. The effect of DFM supplementation on rumen fermentability [3] is shown in **Table 1**.

The results showed that DFM supplementation in feed based on plantation waste in the form of ammoniated palm frond could increase rumen fermentability. The bacterial population increased from 1.61 x 10^9 to 2.35 x 10^9 cell mL-1. These results are following the results of research [1, 9] where the addition of probiotics in the ration can stimulate the development of microbes in the rumen and increase the digestibility of food in livestock. The way yeast works in the rumen can utilize oxygen to ensure anaerobic conditions for rumen bacteria and stimulate specific rumen bacterial populations [25] (**Figure 1**). However, there was a tendency for the bacterial population to decrease in the combination supplementation of three types of DFM (P7). It was suspected that there was an accumulation of rumen microbial

Treatments	Parameters		
	VFA (mM)	NH_3 (mM)	Bacteria population (cell mL^{-1})
P0	108.35^{e}	12.28^{d}	1.61×10^{9e}
P1	130.69^{ab}	14.97^{ab}	2.49×10^{9ab}
P2	125.10^{cd}	14.47^{ab}	2.37×10^{9bc}
P3	123.24^{cd}	13.73^{bc}	2.40×10^{9bc}
P4	126.97^{bc}	15.25^{a}	2.41×10^{9bc}
P5	132.55^{a}	15.75^{a}	2.55×10^{9a}
P6	121.38^{d}	13.06^{cd}	2.35×10^{9c}
P7	121.38^{d}	12.78^{cd}	1.93×10^{9c}
SE	1.806	0.425	3.33

Source: Suryani et al., 2016, DOI: 10.3923/pjn.2017.599.604
Numbers followed by different lowercase letters in the same column (a, b, c, d, and e) were significantly different ($P < 0.05$), SC: Saccharomyces cerevisiae, AO: Aspergillus oryzae, BA: Bacillus amilolyquifaciens, P0: Ammoniated palm fronds, P1: P0 + SC (1%), P2: P0 + AO (1%), P3: P0 + BA (1%), P4: P0 + SC (0.5%) + AO (0.5%), P5: P0 + SC (0.5%) + BA (0.5%), P6: P0 + AO (0.5%) + BA (0.5%), P7: P0 + SC (0.3%) + AO (0.3%) + BA (0.3%), supplementation of DFM % on dry matter basis;

Table 1.
Supplementation of DFM in ammoniated palm fronds on fermentability and bacteria population in vitro.

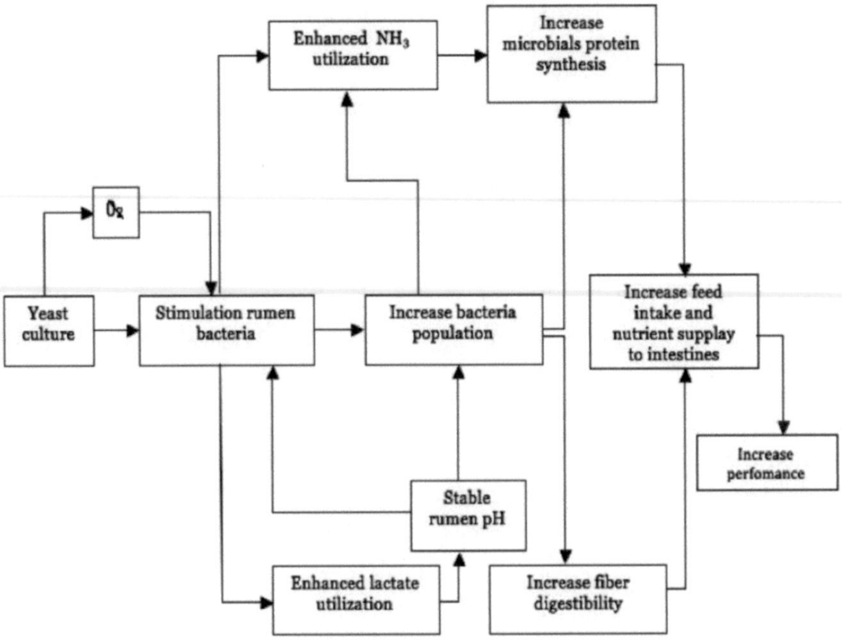

Figure 1.
Mode of action DFM in the rumen.

growth so that bacteria in the rumen competed in digesting feed. The total NH3 and VFA concentrations increased from 12.28 mM to 14.28 mM and 108.35 mM to 125.90 mM. Desnoyers *et al.*, [26] stated that yeast supplementation could increase the concentration of VFA (2.1 mmol L-1) and decrease the concentration of lactate.

Furthermore, DFM fungal *A. oryzae* can reduce oxygen in the rumen [27]. This situation was followed by increased ammonia and lactic acid utilization so that the rumen pH was stable. Anaerobic conditions and stable rumen pH allow more optimal microbial protein synthesis so that the total population of rumen bacteria increases and the digestibility of crude fiber increases. Increased digestibility of crude fiber will increase the consumption and supply of nutrients to the intestines, so that it is expected to increase the overall response of livestock production. Meanwhile, *B. amylolyquifaciens* DFM can produce cellulase enzymes [28], so when yeast is combined with fungal or bacterial DFM, it can increase rumen fermentation with high VFA results. The increase in rumen fermentability was also followed by dry matter and organic matter digestibility which increased from 47.5% (without DFM) to 51.55% (with DFM) and 48.89% to 52.41% [3]. DFM *S. cerevisiae* can be used individually or in combination with *A. oryzae* or *B. amylolyquifaciens*. However, when viewed from the average value produced, the *S. cerevisiae* + *B. amylolyquifaciens* combination gave the best rumen digestibility and fermentability results. This is because *S. cerevisiae* can produce growth factors for microbial growth from organic acids, B vitamins, and amino acids to stimulate rumen microbial activity and development [29]. A brief diagram illustrating the working principle of DFM in the rumen. It can be seen in **Figure 1** [25] modified.

Yeast culture uses oxygen to metabolize feed particles into sugars and oligosaccharides to produce peptides and amino acids as end products used by bacteria. Most rumen microorganisms are anaerobic, so the utilization of oxygen by yeast culture will increase the optimum conditions in the rumen. These conditions will protect the anaerobic rumen bacteria from damage by O2. They created better conditions for the growth of cellulolytic bacteria so that the number of cellulolytic bacteria increases and improves digestion in the rumen [30].

Yeast activity as DFM can regulate rumen biological activity by stimulating lactic acid utilization and reducing ammonia production, so that rumen pH is stable and increases nutrient absorption and VFA profile [31]. Supplementation can support livestock productivity by increasing intestinal development, mucosal immunity, nutrient absorption, and inhibiting pathogenic bacteria. This will have an impact on improving livestock health and performance [32].

2.2 Effect virgin coconut oils on methane gas concentration

In another study, to streamline the digestive process in the rumen, Suryani *et al.*, [3] continued the best DFM results from the 1st stage of the experiment to be combined with methane emission reducers. Virgin coconut oil (VCO), rich in MCFA, is used to reduce methane emissions. VCO is oil produced from fresh coconuts. VCO contains lauric acid (C12:0), which effectively suppresses methanogenic bacteria and rumen protozoa [5]. The VCO used in this study contained lauric acid (C12: 0) 51.95% [21] (**Figure 2**).

The purpose of this experiment is to get the best VCO level combined with the best type of DFM stage 1 on ammoniated palm fronds. The three VCO levels tested were 2, 3, and 4% DM. The two best types of DFM from stage 1 used as controls were *S. cerevisiae* and *S. cerevisiae* + *B. amyloliquifaciens* 1% DM. Experiments were carried out *in vitro* according to the method [24].

The effect of combined VCO and DFM supplementation on methane gas concentration and rumen protozoa population *in vitro* on ammoniated palm frond-based feed can be seen in **Table 2**, **Figures 3** and **4**.

The results of the orthogonal polynomial test show a quadratic relationship ($P < 0.05$) between the level of VCO (X, %) and the concentration of methane gas in the rumen (Y, mM) with the equation y = 1.2682x2–7.3169 + 22.281 and the coefficient of determination $R^2 = 0.98137$ (**Figure 3**).

Based on the orthogonal polynomial test, methane gas concentration at the level of 2% VCO addition with DFM *S. cerevisiae* and *S. cerevisiae* + *B. amyloliquifaciens* decreased by 48.11% and 43.67%, respectively. The addition of a 3% VCO level also decreased methane gas concentration compared to without supplementation and resulted in an average of 11.87 mM and 12.58 mM. The decrease in methane gas concentration occurs because VCO is rich in MCFA, mainly lauric acid (C12:0) (**Figure 2**), which is effective in suppressing methanogenic bacteria and rumen protozoa [5]. Lauric acid is the most toxic to protozoa [33] and is the most potent antiprotozoal that inhibits ciliated protozoa's growth and activity (mainly *Entodinium spp.)* [22]. The decrease in ciliate protozoa population due to defaunation causes a decrease in the symbiosis

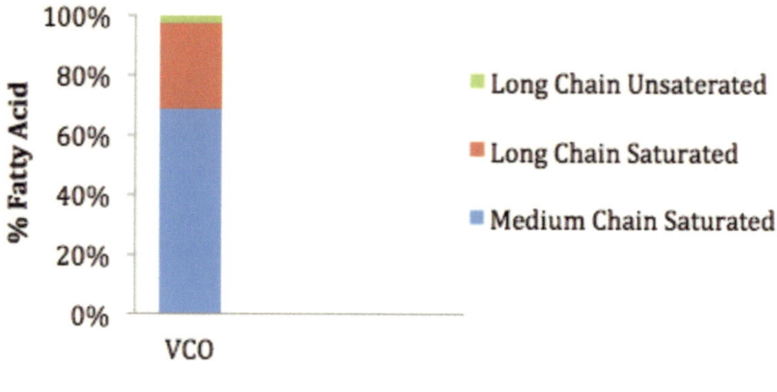

Figure 2.
Fatty acid composition of VCO.

Treatments	CH_4 (ml/g DM)	Protozoa (cell/mL-1)
P1: SC 1% + 0% VCO	21.74 ± 1.16	7.08 x 10^4 ± 0.23
P2: SC 0.5% + BA 0.5% + 0% VCO	22.94 ± 0.84	7.23 x 10^4 ± 0.36
P3: SC 1% + 2% VCO	11.78 ± 0.62	1.92 x 10^4 ± 0.09
P4: SC 0.5% + BA 0.5% + 2% VCO	12.92 ± 0.22	2.23 x 10^4 ± 0.09
P5: SC 1% + 3% VCO	11.87 ± 0.79	1.97 x 10^4 ± 0.09
P6: SC 0.5% + BA 0.5% + 3% VCO	12.58 ± 0.15	2.65 x 10^4 ± 0.15
P7: SC 1% + 4% VCO	12.75 ± 0.93	3.38 x 10^4 ± 0.09
P8: SC 0.5% + BA 0.5% + 4% VCO	13.49 ± 0.09	3.28 x 10^4 ± 0.15

Note. Substrate based on Ammoniated palm frond treated with 6% urea, DFM supplementation and VCO level on dry matter basis, SC: Saccharomyces cerevisiae, AO: Aspergillus oryzae BA: Bacillus amilolyquifaciens, VCO: Virgin coconut oils;

Table 2.
Production of methane (CH_4) and protozoa population from the fermentation of ammoniated palm fronds in vitro in the rumen for each DFM type level and VCO levels.

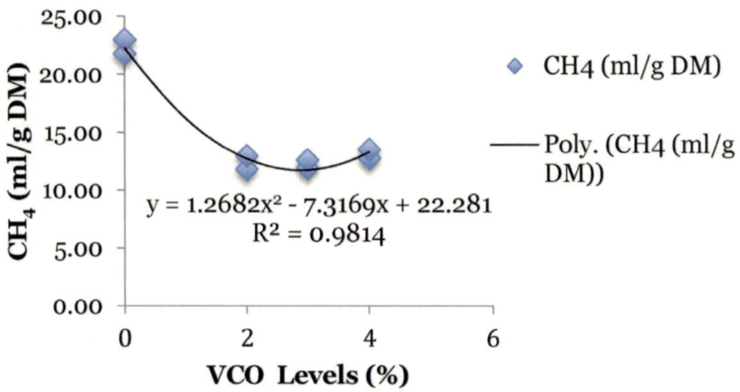

Figure 3.
The relationship between DFM + VCO levels and methane production from rumen fermentation of ammoniated palm frond during 48 hours incubation.

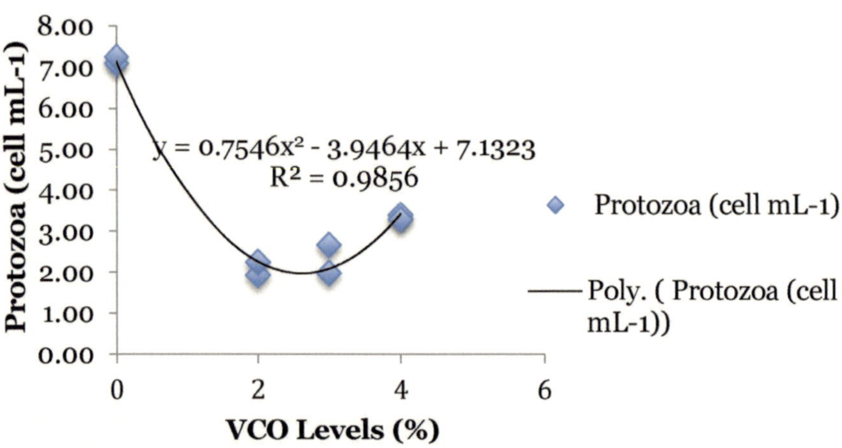

Figure 4.
The relationship between DFM + VCO levels and the population of protozoa produced by fermenting the rumen of ammoniated palm frond during 48 hours of incubation.

between ciliate protozoa and methanogens, thereby reducing the availability of hydrogen for methane formation [17].

Furthermore, Dohmet *et al.*, [33] reported that lauric acid (C12:0) and myristic acid (C14:0) could reduce methanogenesis in the rumen and significantly reduce total methanogenic bacteria. This result is also supported by Machmuller *et al.*, [20]. The effect of coconut oil supplementation is to reduce methane by inhibiting the metabolic activity of archaea methanogens directly in the rumen.

Supplementation of *S. cerevisiae* and VCO DFM at all levels (P3, P5, and P7) can reduce methane cocntentration better than the combination of DFM *S. cerevisiae* + *B. amyloliquifaciens* and VCO at all levels (P4, P6, and P8). This indicates that when *S. cerevisiae* type DFM combined with VCO can support a decrease in methane concentration in rumen fermentation activity, this is also suspected because *S. cerevisiae* as DFM also can reduce methane. *Yeast* supplementation can also stimulate acetogenins to compete for hydrogen with methanogens, thereby reducing methane emissions [34].

The results of the orthogonal polynomial test give a quadratic relationship between the VCO level (X, %) and the protozoa population (Y, cell/mL-1), the Eq. Y = 0.7546x2–3.9464x + 7.1323 and the coefficient of determination (R2) = 0.98564 is shown on **Figure 4**. The average population of protozoa with the addition of VCO in the rumen can be seen in **Table 3**.

Based on the orthogonal polynomial test, the protozoa population decreased with VCO supplementation. Supplementation of 2% and 3% VCO (P3,P4,P5,P6) on palm fronds with the addition of DFM *S. cerevisiae* and *S. cerevisiae* + *B. amyloliquifaciens* reduced the protozoa population by 72.88%, 69.15%, 72, 17 and 63.32%, respectively. This result was also followed by a decrease in methane gas concentartion in this treatment. Protozoa populations are closely related to rumen methane production [35]. 7 to 37% of methanogens live in symbiosis with protozoa in the rumen [5]. The results of this combination of DFM and VCO supplementation resulted in a decrease in the percentage of protozoa population, which was the same as that obtained by Kongmun *et al.* [36] that the protozoa decreased 68–75% by

Variables	Treatments				SE
	A	B	C	D	
DM Intake (kg day^{-1})	3.16^a	3.01^b	2.99^b	2.57^c	0.143
DM/$BW^{0.75}$ (g kg^{-1} $b.wt.^{0.75}$ d^{-1})	79.94^a	75.68^{ab}	74.24^{ab}	67.36^b	1.790
OM Intake (kg/h/d)	3.93^a	3.74^b	3.72^b	3.19^c	0.017
OM /$BW^{0.75}$ (g kg^{-1} $b.wt.^{0.75}$ d^{-1})	99.28^a	97.14^a	93.98^a	83.65^b	1.504
ADG (kg day^{-1})	0.53^c	0.63^b	0.63^b	0.71^a	0.007
Feed Efficiency (%)	16.96^c	20.84^b	21.34^b	27.77^a	0.311
Methane production (L day^{-1})	109.01^c	103.27^b	102.61^b	86.52^a	0.501
Nitrogen intake (g day^{-1})	59.20^a	56.34^b	55.96^b	47.84^c	0.815
Nitrogen retention (g day^{-1})	50.51^a	47.99^a	47.16^a	37.23^b	0.797

Source: Suryani et al., 2017,http://dx.doi.org/10.3923/ pjn.2017.599.604.
Numbers followed by different lowercase letters (a, b, c) in the same row are significantly different (P < 0.05), A: 100% Complete feed, B: A + 1% SC, C: A + 0.5% SC + 0.5% BA, D: A + 2% VCO + 1% SC. DM: Dry matter, OM: Organic matter, BW: Body weight, ADG: Average daily gain, SC: Saccharomyces cerevisiae, BA: Bacillus amilolyquifaciens, VCO: Virgin coconut oils;

Table 3.
Effect of DFM and VCO supplementation on consumption, ADG, efficiency, and methane production of Bali cattle.

supplementing with 7% coconut oil. Furthermore, this result is greater than that obtained [37] that coconut oil and lauric acid supplementation reduced the protozoan population by up to 40%.

Meanwhile, total protozoa (especially *Entodinium spp*) decreased by 96% due to lauric acid supplementation compared to myrystic acid on a concentrate rich substrate [38]. This indicates that DFM supplementation in high-fiber feeds such as palm oil plantation waste plays an important role in modifying the rumen ecosystem so that the addition of VCO at the right level can reduce the concentration of methane and protozoa without reducing nutrient degradation. From the results of this study, it is recommended that 2% VCO be used for cattle *in vivo* because levels 3 and 4% give almost the same average results.

In other studies, Suryani *et al* [24] continued the experimental *in vitro* studies of stages I and II into a complete ration formulation based on ammoniated palm fronds prepared with a TDN content of 63.28%. *In vivo* tests were carried out using 16 Bali cattle to determine the effect of adding DFM *S. cerevisiae*, *S. cerevisiae* + *B. amyloliquifaciens*, and *S. cerevisiae* + 2% VCO on livestock productivity. Blood samples were collected to determine the effect of DFM and VCO supplementation on the blood profile. Blood samples were taken once before the cattle were fed in the morning (fasting). Blood samples were taken through the jugular vein using a 10 ml capacity syringe and placed in a vacutainer. Blood serum was separated using centrifugation at 3000 rpm for 10 minutes. Analysis of glucose levels, total protein, urea, BUN, albumin, triglycerides, total cholesterol, HDL, and LDL was carried out using the HumaStar 80® Auto Analyzer. A statistical test was carried out to determine the effect of treatment on the observed parameters, using a variance according to the design used. If there was a significant effect, it was continued with Duncan's test [39].

The effect of DFM and VCO supplementation on Bali cattle on performance and methane gas production [21] is shown in **Table 3**.

DFM and VCO supplementation decreased methane production by 5.26, 5.87, and 20.63% respectively. The highest ration efficiency was in DFM *S. cerevisiae* + 2% VCO supplementation, followed by ADG at 0.70 (kg/h/d) and decreased methane production by 20.63% [21]. DFM yeast was reported to have the ability to reduce methane production by 28% [40]. Yeast supplementation could also stimulate acetogens to compete for hydrogen with methanogens, thereby reducing methane emissions [41]. With reduced methane production in the rumen, it can increase feed energy, which positively affects livestock performance. This can be seen from the decrease in DM and OM consumption but can increase Efficiency and ADG. The digestibility of DM, OM, NDF, ADF, Cellulose, and TDN also increased with DFM supplementation and the combination of DFM *S. cerevisiae* + VCO [21]. The mechanism of DFM can reduce methane production, presumably because DFM microorganisms can stimulate the development of rumen microbes in digesting feed so that fermentation of carbohydrates in the rumen results in high production of propionate. In the rumen, propionate production requires H2 bound to glucose which is described in the following equation.

$$\mathrm{C6H12O6} + \mathrm{2H2} \rightarrow \mathrm{2CH3}CH\mathrm{2COOH} + \mathrm{4H2}$$

Therefore, to reduce hydrogen production to methane, hydrogen must be switched to propionate production via lactate or fumarate [42]. H2 and CO2 are substrates used to form methane. According to Wilkie [43] the role of hydrogen in the methane production process is as a source of electrons, so the low level of H2 in the rumen is an indication of activity using H2 to reduce CO2 to CH. In addition, to form one mole of CH4 requires four moles of H2. The rate of H2 utilization is four times the rate of methane production so that H2 in the rumen never accumulates. The following is the stoichiometry of the carbohydrate fermentation reaction in producing methane gas in the rumen:

$$4H2 + CO2 \rightarrow CH4 + 2H2O$$

The effect of DFM and VCO supplementation on Bali cattle on blood profile can be seen in **Table 4**.

The results showed that DFM and VCO supplementation had a very significant effect ($p < 0.05$) in reducing cholesterol, LDL and increasing HDL blood levels of Bali cattle. DFM and VCO supplementation had no significant effect ($P > 0.05$) on triglycerides, urea, protein, albumin, and glucose. VCO contains MCFA, which is a saturated fatty acid (**Figure 1**), its addition in the ration if consumed by livestock can help lower cholesterol because of the nature of this fatty acid, which can be absorbed directly by the animal's body so that it does not cause fat accumulation that causes cholesterol. This is supported by Fernando *et al.* [44], which states that MCFA is directly converted into energy in the liver and increases metabolic rate, and reduces fat deposits in the body. MCFA has a very high solubility in water and requires fewer digestive enzymes, making it burnt into energy. MCFA is burned to produce energy and encourages the combustion of LCFA [45]. So there is a significant decrease in the amount of LDL and is followed by an increase in HDL in the blood. The calories contained are also lower than long-chain fatty acids [46]. Reducing fat deposits in the body can lower LDL cholesterol and increase HDL cholesterol [47].

This study can conclude that individual *S. cerevisiae* DFM supplementation and *S. cerevisiae* + *B. amyloliquifaciens* combination can optimize bioprocesses in the rumen. VCO supplementation level of 2% can be used to suppress methane production. Supplementation of *S. cerevisiae* type DFM and 2% VCO level can be considered to optimize bioprocesses in the rumen, increasing performance and reducing methane production in Bali cattle fed complete rations based on ammoniated palm fronds.

Variables	Treatments				SE
	A	B	C	D	
Cholesterol (mg/dl)	137.18^{a}	124.25^{b}	122.00^{b}	108.69^{c}	1.508
Triglycerides (mg/dl)	87.29	89.08	95.70	108.49	3.305
LDL (mg/dl)	76.14^{a}	72.49^{b}	70.43^{b}	67.18^{c}	0.501
HDL (mg/dl)	184.00^{a}	170.07^{b}	168.05^{b}	147.00^{c}	1.814
Urea (mg/dl)	29.42	24.53	24.06	19.53	0.954
Protein (g/dl)	6.17	6.99	7.18	7.66	0.226
Albumin (g/dl	3.13	3.31	3.45	3.56	0.046
Glucose (mg/dl)	70.09	73.75	76.69	80.08	0.679

Numbers followed by different lowercase letters (a, b, c) in the same row are significantly different ($P < 0.05$), A: 100% Complete feed, B: A + 1% SC, C: A + 0.5% SC + 0.5% BA, D: A + 2% VCO + 1% SC. DFM: Direct fed microbials, SC: Saccharomyces cerevisiae, BA: Bacillus amilolyquifaciens, VCO: Virgin coconut oils, LDL: low density lipoprotein, HDL: high density lipoprotein.

Table 4.
Blood profile of complete diet based on ammoniated palm fronds supplemented with DFM and VCO.

3. Effect of different source tannins on methane gas production

Bioactive compounds, including polyphenols, carotenoids, omega-3 fatty acids, vitamins, organic acids, nucleotides, and nucleosides, have attracted significant attention for their role in preventing several chronic diseases in humans. In animal husbandry, especially ruminant nutrition, bioactive plant polyphenolic compounds such as tannins and saponins have been studied extensively for optimizing bioprocesses in the rumen through feed manipulation. Manipulation of feed using tannins as an agent of rumen defaunation is one way to overcome global climate change due to the effects of greenhouse gases, one of which is caused by methane gas from ruminants [18]. Feeds containing tannins will be anti-nutrients that limit livestock production when the crude protein concentration in the feed is high because it can reduce the absorption of amino acids [48]. Tannins can also cause poisoning if consumed by livestock in excess, and there are many *in vitro* and *in vivo* studies that describe the methane inhibitory effect of tannins [19]. The study results Staerfl *et al.* [49] proved that the use of tannins could reduce CH4 emissions by up to 36% in bulls fed grass, corn silage, and concentrate rations. Not many studies have explored the use of tannins in feed based on plantation waste. Therefore, the authors are interested in conducting a series of experiments using tannins from different sources. Plant bioactive compounds used are tannins derived from *gambir leaves waste* (GLW) and obtained from two different sources or areas, namely GLW Payahkumbuh and Painan. GLW was added at different levels (10, 15, 20%) to the ammonium palm midrib substrate with the addition of 4% urea [50]. Experiments were carried out *in vitro* and *in vivo*.

In another *in vitro* study in the same group, the authors also tried to compare *Gliricidia sepium* in animal feed based on rice straw plantation waste [51]. *Gliricidia sepium* is a bioactive plant compound containing thick tannins and saponins capable of modifying the number of rumen microbes such as archaea, protozoa, and fibriolytic bacteria that affect the fermentative process and production of methane gas [52]. The study was conducted *in vitro*. Complete feed is prepared based on ammoniated rice straw. Three levels of *Gliricidia sepium* tested were 10, 20, and 30% DM basis. The study results, the effect of different sources and levels of tannins on dry matter digestibility (DM), organic matter (OM), methane gas concentration, protozoa, and bacteria can be seen in **Table 5**.

The results showed that different sources and doses of tannins proved to have different effects on decreasing methane production [50]. The *in vitro* study results showed that supplementation of 15% GLW and 10% GLW, which had a total tannin concentration of 12.5 and 15.6% dry matter, respectively, could reduce methane gas concentration by 53% and 45% compared to control. The decrease in methane gas was followed by a decrease in the protozoa population by 53.89% compared to control. Different levels and sources of GLW had no significant effect ($P > 0.05$) on the total bacterial population. However, there is a tendency for the bacterial population to increase as the population of protozoa and methane decreases. Tannins decrease methane production by reducing methanogenic bacteria and protozoa [53]. Furthermore, it was reported that condensed tannins extracted from different plants had different effects on rumen fermentation characteristics. This is because it is associated with different chemical structures and molecular weights [54, 55]. Condensed tannins extracted from different plants have varied activities in binding carbohydrates and proteins [56].

Furthermore, the *in vitro* results of the addition of GLW as a source of tannins were tested *in vivo* on three Simmental cattle [12] with a weight ranging between 179 and 190 kg using the BSL design. The results showed that two sources of tannin levels could increase nutrient digestibility but had no effect on protein digestibility,

Treatments	DM (%)	OM (%)	Protozoa population (cell mL-1)	CH_4 (ml/g DM)	VFA Total (mM)	A: P Ratio
T0	48.45[b]	51.34[b]	11.43 x 10[4a]	27.22[a]	71.00[b]	3.98[a]
B1	51.59[ab]	54.17[ab]	2.3 x 10[4c]	23.64[ab]	83.70[ab]	2.70[c]
B2	52.09[a]	57.30[a]	1.4 x 10[4c]	12.67[c]	95.78[a]	3.52[ab]
B3	50.93[ab]	53.15[ab]	4.8 x 10[4b]	13.14[c]	65.94[b]	3.38[ab]
C1	51.08[ab]	54.16[ab]	4.7 x 10[4a]	15.13[c]	75.49[ab]	2.58[b]
C2	50.69[ab]	52.83[ab]	9.3 x 10[4b]	17.12[c]	79.40[ab]	3.65[a]
C3	48.65[b]	51.04[b]	8.8 x 10[4a]	21.90[b]	62.44[b]	3.40[b]
A	58,83[c]	59.50c	6.3 x 10[5a]	22.72[a]	72.00	2.14[b]
B	62.5[b]	63.72b	5.8 x 10[5b]	21.46[b]	74.25	1.50[a]
C	66.33[a]	68.66a	4.9 x 10[5c]	16.27[c]	75.45	1.70[a]
D	68.54[a]	69.50a	4.7 x 10[5c]	14.14[c]	76.8	1.33[a]

Sources: Ningrat et al., 2017; DOI: 10.3923/ajas.2017.47.53; Zain et al., 2020; DOI:10.18517/ijaseit.10.2.11242. Different superscripts in the same column highly significant effect (p < 0.05), T0: Oil palm frond ammoniated previously treated by 4% urea as control, B1: A + 10% GLW Payakumbuh, B2: A + 15% GLW Payakumbuh, B3: A + 20% GLW Payakumbuh, C1: A + 10% GLW Painan, C2: A + 15% GLW Painan, C3: A + 20% GLW Painan. A: 40% ammoniated rice straw +60% concentrate, B: 40% ammoniated rice straw +50% concentrate + 10% Gliricidia sepium, C: 40% ammoniated rice straw +40% concentrate +20% Gliricidia sepium, D: 40% ammoniated rice straw +30%, DM: Dry matter, OM: Organic matter, VFA: Volatile fatty acid, GLW: gambir leaves waste;

Table 5.
Effect different sources and doses of tannin on dry matter (DM), organic matter (OM), protozoa population, methane (CH_4) production, VFA total, and acetate: Propionate ratio based on agriculture by-product as feed in the rumen.

urinary allantoin, and nutrient consumption. The addition of 15% GLW tannins and 10% GLW Painan in the ration significantly increased ADG and decreased methane production compared to controls, namely 0.65, 0.90, 0.92 kg/day, and 2.48, 1.28, 1.26 MJ/day [12]. Saponins contained in GLW can increase the efficiency of rumen fermentation through the mechanism of reducing the population of protozoa [57]. The decrease in the protozoa population will cause the availability of H2 for methanogens to decrease [58]. The reduction in protozoa population supports stabilization of rumen pH and an increase in the population of cellulolytic microorganisms. Thus, decreased methanogenesis will increase the efficiency of digestibility in high fiber rations and livestock performance.

The addition of *G. sepium* in the diet resulted in a decrease in methane production and the highest protozoa population at the levels of 20 and 30%, namely 12.67, 13.16 mM, and 4.9 x 105, 4.7 x 105 cell/ml *in vitro*. However, there was no significant difference (P > 0.05) between the two levels. The treatment had no significant effect (p > 0.05) on total VFA, acetate, butyrate, valerate + isovalerate + isobutyrate. Acetate propionate ratio decreased respectively to 2.14, 1.50, 1.70, 1.33. The propionate concentration increased by 43.87% compared to the control, and there was no significant difference (P > 0.05) between levels of gliricidia addition [51]. Plant bioactive compound *Gliricidia sepium* contains tannins and saponins, which effectively reduce the population of protozoa and methane production. The feed used in this study was based on agricultural waste with high fiber content. In addition to saponin's structure, which can affect protozoa's activity, the type of feed given can also affect the fermentation process in the rumen [59]. In the study Zain *et al.*, [51] the types of protozoa that survived the addition of *Gliricidia sepium* were not identified. However, the results obtained showed that the saponins and tannins in *Gliricidia sepium* could inhibit certain types of protozoa that cause a decrease in protozoa population in the rumen. The decrease in methane production and the protozoa population with 20 and 30% *Gliricidia sepium* can increase the digestibility of dry matter and organic matter produced [51].

The potential of plant bioactive compounds such as tannins and saponins as defaunation agents and reducing methane emissions can be combined with direct-fed microbes. There is not much literature on decreasing methane production that combines the two in *vivo* studies. *In vitro* studies Arowolo *et al.* [60] stated that there is a synergistic effect between probiotics and plant bioactive compounds simultaneously to stabilize the rumen fermentation process and reduce methane production. However, it still requires further studies at the *in vivo* level. Based on these results, Ningrat *et al.* [61] conducted a test of *Gliricidia sepium* and DFM *S. cerevisiae* supplementation to improve the performance of Simmental cattle while reducing methane gas production. It was found that the combined supplementation of 1% SC and 15% *Gliricidia sepium* significantly increased the digestibility of DM, and OM, ADG, and methane gas production compared to *S. cerevisiae* and *Gliricidia sepium* supplementation individually. The decrease in methane production with the addition of SC, GLW, and the combination of *S. cerevisiae* + *Gliricidia sepium* respectively 1.42, 1.35, and 1.02 MJ.day-1 [61]. These results prove that yeast culture can work synergistically when combined with reducing agents. Emissions of methane plant bioactive compounds such as tannins and saponins. Tannin compounds inhibit the activity of methanogens [62] and can defaunate [63]. Pineiro-Vazquez *et al.* [64] reported the results of an *in vivo* evaluation showing the effect of 80% Leucaena sp. (21% condensed tannins) in the diet composition was able to reduce methane emissions by 61.3% without affecting nutrient intake and VFA production in the Bos taurus × Bos indicus cross.

4. Conclusion

In conclusion, the overall reduction in methane production in agriculture by-products as feed-based beef cattle can be made by improving feed quality through a combination of processing techniques and efforts to optimize bioprocesses in the rumen, which include supplementation of feed additives such as direct-fed microbials, methanogenesis inhibitors and plant bioactive compounds. Supplementation of DFM type *S. cerevisiae* 1% combined with 2% VCO can reduce methane production by 20.36% and increase ADG by 0.70 kg/day in Bali cattle. Plant bioactive compounds, especially tannins from *Gliricidia sepium*, can be used up to 15% in amniotic palm frond-based rations. *Gliricidia sepium*, which contains tannins and saponins at levels of 20 and 30% dry matter in complete rations, can also reduce methane, protozoa population and increase livestock performance. The combination of DFM *S. cerevisiae* and *Gliricidia sepium* can also be used to reduce methane gas production in Simmental cattle fed complete feed based on 46.61% amniotic palm fronds compared to controls.

Acknowledgements

Thank to the Ministry of Research and Technology, and Andalas University that providing grants to support the research.

Author details

Mardiati Zain[1]*, Rusmana Wijaya Setia Ningrat[1], Heni Suryani[2] and Novirman Jamarun[1]

1 Faculty of Animal Science, Universitas Andalas, Padang, Indonesia

2 Faculty of Animal Science, Universitas Jambi, Jambi, Indonesia

*Address all correspondence to: mardiati@ansci.unand.ac.id

References

[1] Zain M, Jamarun N, Arnim A, Ningrat RWS, Herawaty R. Effect of yeast (*Saccharomyces cerevisiae*) on fermentability, microbial population, and digestibility of low-quality roughage *in vitro*. Arch. Zootech. 2011: 14: 51-58.

[2] Herawaty R, Jamarun N, Zain M, Arnim and Ningrat RWS. Effect of supplementation Saccharomyces cerevisiae and Leucaena leucocephala on low quality roughage feed in beef cattle diet. Pak. J. Nutr. 2013: 12: 182-184. Doi: 10.3923/pjn.2013.182.184

[3] Suryani H, Zain M, Ningrat RWS, Jamarun N. Supplementation of *Direct Fed Microbials* (DFM) on *in vitro* fermentability and degradability of ammoniated palm frond. Pak. J. Nutr. 2016: 15: 90-95. https://scialert.net/abstract/?doi=pjn.2016.89.94

[4] Mustangwa T, Edward IE, Topps JH and Peterson GFM. The effect of dierty inclusion yeast culture (*Yea-Saac*) on pattern of rumen fermentation, food intake and growth of intensively fed bulls. Anim. Prod. 1992: 55: 35-40. DOI: https://doi.org/10.1017/S0003356100037247

[5] Machmuller A, Soliva CR, and Kreuzer M. Effect of Coconut Oil and Defaunation Treatment on Methanogenesis in sheeep. J. Reprod. Nuter. Dev. 2003: 43: 41-55. https://doi.org/10.1051/rnd:2003005

[6] Brashears MM, Amezquita A and Jaroni D. Lactic acid bacteria and their uses in animal feeding to improve food safety. Adv. Food Nut. Res. 2005: 50:1- 31. DOI: 10.1016/S1043-4526(05)50001-9

[7] Musa HH, We SL, Zhu CH, Seri HI and Zhu GQ. The Potential Benefits of Probiotics in Animal Production And Health. J. Anim. Vet. Adv. 2009: 8: 313-321.

[8] Oyetayo VO, and Oyetayo FL. Potential of Probiotics as Biotherapeutic Agents Targeting the Innate Immune System. Afr. J. Biotech. 2005: 4: 123-127.https://doi.org/10.5897/AJB2005.000-3025

[9] Zain M, Jurnida R, Khasrad and Erpomen. In vitro Fermentation Characteristics of Palm Oil By products Which is Supplemented with Growth Factor Rumen Microbes. Pakistan Journal of Nutrition. 2015: 14 (9): 625-628.: 10.3923/pjn.2015.625.628

[10] Lynch HA and Martin SA. Effect of *Saccharomyces cerevisiae* culture and *Saccharomyces cerevisiae* live cells on in vitro mixed ruminal mircoorganism fermentation. J. Dairy. Sci. 2002: 85: 2603-2608. https://doi.org/10.3168/jds.S0022-0302(02)74345-2

[11] Zain, M. N. Jamarun, and Nurhaita. Effect of Sulfur Supplementation on in vitro Fermentability and Degradability of Ammoniated Rice Straw. Pakistan Journal of Nutrition. 2010: 9 (5): 413-415. DOI: 10.3923/pjn.2010.413.415

[12] Ningrat RWS, Zain M, Erpomen and Suryani H. Effects of supplementation of different sources of tannins on nutrient digestibility, methane production and daily weight gain of beef cattle fed on ammoniated oil palm frond based diet. Inter. J. of Zoological Research. 2018. 14 (1): 8 – 13. DOI: 10.3923/ijzr.2018.8.13

[13] Steinfeld H, Gerber P, Wassenaar T, Castel V, rosales M, de Haan C. Livestock's long shadow,. FAO, Rome 2006. http://www.fao.org/docrep/010/a0701e/a0701e00.HTM

[14] Miller TL, Wolin MJ, Hongxue Z, and Bryant MP. Characteristics of Methanogens Isolated from Bovine Rumen. Applied and Environmental Microbiology. American Sociey for

Microbiology. 2002: 51: 201-202. https://doi.org/10.1128/AEM.51.1.201-202.1986

[15] Moss AR, Jouany JP, and Newbold J. Methane production by ruminants: its contribution to global warming. Ann. Zootech. 2000: 49: 231-253. https://doi.org/10.1051/animres:2000119

[16] Dohme F, Machmuller A, Esterman BL, Pfister P, Wasserfallen A, and Kreuzer M. The role of the rumen protozoa fo methane suppression caused by coconut oil. Letters in Applied Microbiology. 1999. 29: 187-192. https://doi.org/10.1046/j.1365-2672.1999.00614.x

[17] Jordan E, Kenny D, Hawkins M, Malone R, Lovett DK, and O'Mara FP. Effect oy refined soy oil or whole soybeans on intake, methane output, and performance of young bulls. J.Anim.Sci. 2006: 84: 2418-2425. DOI: 10.2527/jas.2005-354

[18] Makkar HPS. Effect and fate of tannins in ruminant animals, adaptation to tannins, andstrategies to overcome detrimental e ects o eeding tannin-rich feeds. Small Ruminant Res. 2003: 49: 241-256. https://doi.org/10.1016/S0921-4488(03)00142-1

[19] Jayanegara A, Leiber F and Kreuzer M. Meta-analysis of the relationship between dietary tannin level and methane formation in ruminants from in vivo and in vitro experiments. Journal of Animal Physiology and Animal Nutrition. 2012: 96:365-375. https://doi.org/10.1111/j.1439-0396.2011.01172.x

[20] Machmuller, A. Medium chain fatty acids and their potential to reduce methanogenesis in dosmetic ruminants. Agric. Ecosyst. Environ. 2006: 112: 107-114. https://doi.org/10.1016/j.agee.2005.08.010

[21] Suryani H, Zain M, Ningrat RWS, Jamarun N. Effect of dietary supplementation based on an ammoniated palm frond with direct fed microbials and virgin coconut oil on the growth performance and methane production of Bali cattle. Pak. J. Nutr. 2017: 16: 599-604. http://dx.doi.org/10.3923/ pjn.2017.599.604

[22] Soliva CR, Meile L, Hindrichsen IK, Kreuzer M, and Machmuller. Myristic acid supports the immediate inhibitory effect of lauric acid on ruminal methanogens and methane release. Anaerobe. 2004: 10: 269-276. https://doi.org/10.1016/j.anaerobe.2004.06.003

[23] Beauchemin KA, McGinn SM, Martinez TF, and McAlliste TA. Use of condensed tannin extract from quebracho trees to reduce methane emission from cattle. J Anim Sci. 2007: 85:1990-1996. DOI: 10.2527/jas.2006-686

[24] Tilley JMA and Terry RA. A two stage technique for the in vitro digestion of forage crops. Journal of British Grassland Society. 1963: 18: 104 – 111. https://doi.org/10.1111/j.1365-2494.1963.tb00335.x

[25] Yoon IK and Stern MD. Influence of directed fed microbials on ruminal microbial fermentation and performance of ruminants. A Review. Asian-Aust. J. Anim. Sci. 1995: 8: 535 – 555

[26] Desnoyers M, Giger-Reverdin S, Bertin G, Duvaux-Ponter C and Sauvant D. Meta-Analysis of The Influence Of *Saccharomyces Cerevisiae* Supple- mentation on Ruminal Parameters And Milk Production of Ruminant. J. Dairy. Sci. 2009: 92: 1620-1632. DOI: 10.3168/jds.2008-1414

[27] Seo JK, Kim JS, Kim MH, Upadhaya SD, Kam DK, Ha JK. Direct-fed microbials for ruminant animals. Asian Australasian Journal of Animal Sciences. 2010: 23: 1657-1667. Doi: 10.5713/AJAS.2010.R.08

[28] Wizna., H. Abbas, Y. Rizal, A. Dharma dan I. P. Kompiang. Selection and identification of cellulase-producing bacteria isolated from the litter of mountain and swampy forest. Microbiology Indonesia Journal, December. 2007: 1(3): 135-139. Doi: https://doi.org/10.5454/mi.1.3.7

[29] Wiedmeier, R.D., M.J. Arambel, and J.L. Walters. Effect of yeast culture and *aspergillus oryzae* fermentation extract on ruminal characteristics and nutrient digestibility. J. Dairy Sci. 1987: 70:2063-2068. https://doi.org/10.3168/jds.S0022-0302(87)80254-0

[30] Jouany JP. Twenty years of research and now more relevant than ever the coming of age of yeast cultures in ruminant diets. In: Responding to a Changing Agricultural Landscape. Alltech's European, Middle Eastern and African Lecture Tour. 2001. 44-69 p.

[31] Wang Y, Wu X, Chen J, Amin R, Lu M, Bayana B, Zhao J, Murray CK, Hamblin MR, Hooper DC, and Dai T. Antimicrobial blue light in-activation of gram-negative pathogens in biofilms: in vitro and in vivo studies. The J. of Infectious Dieasis. 2016. 213 (9): 1380-1387. Doi: 10.1093/infdis/jiw070

[32] Suryani H, Zain M, Jamarun N, Ningrat RWS. The role of Direct Fed Microbials (DFM) *Saccharomyces cerevisiae* and *Aspergillus oryzae* on ruminant productivity: a Review. Jurnal Peternakan Indonesia. 2015: 17: 27-37. https://doi.org/10.25077/jpi.17.1.27-37.2015

[33] Dohme F, Machmuller A, Wasserfallen A and Kreuzer M. Ruminal methanogenesis as influence y individual fatty acids supplemented to complete ruminant diets. Lett. Applied Microbiol. 2001: 32: 47-51. DOI: 10.1046/j.1472-765x.2001.00863.x

[34] Chaucheyras F, Fonty G, Bertin G, Salmon JM and Gouet P. Effects of a strain of *Saccharomyces cerevisiae* (Levucell SC), a microbial additive for ruminants, on lactate metabolism *in vitro*. Can. J. Microbiol. 1995: 42: 927-933. DOI: 10.1139/m96-119

[35] Guyader J, Eugene M, Noziere P, Morgavi DP, Doreau SE, and McSweeney CS. Effect of tea saponin on methanogenesis, microbial community structure and expression of mcrA gene, in cultures of rumen microorganism. Lett. Appl. Microbiol. 2008: 47: 421-426. DOI: 10.1111/j.1472-765X.2008.02459.x

[36] Kongmun P, Wanapat M, Pakdee P, Navanukraw C, and Yu Z. Manipulation of Rumen Fermentation and Ecology of Swamp Buffalo by Coconut Oil and Garlic Powder Supplementation. J. Liv. Sci. 2010: 01315. https://doi.org/10.1016/j.livsci.2010.06.131

[37] Faciola AP and Broderick GA. Effect of feeding lauric acid or coconut oil on ruminal protozoa numbers, fermentation pattern, digestion, omasal nutrient flow, and milk production in dairy cow. J. Dairy Sci. 2014: 97: 5088-5100.doi.10.3168/jds.2013-7653. https://doi.org/10.3168/jds.2013-7653

[38] Hristov AN, Callaway TR, C. Lee, SE and Dowd SE. Rumen Bacterial, Archaeal, and Fungal Diversity of Dairy Cows in Response to Ingestion of Lauric or Myristic Acid. J. Anim. Sci. 2012: 90: 4449-4457. DOI: 10.2527/jas.2011-4624

[39] Wiliam P E V. Understanding the biochemical mode of action of yeast culture. In. Biotechnology in the Feed Industry. LYONS, T.P. (Ed.). Alltech Techinical Publication, Nicholasville. Kentucky. 1988. 79- 100 p.

[40] Steel RGD, Torrie JH. Principles and procedures of statistics. McGraw-Hill Inc. 1993. New York, USA

[41] Mwenya B, Santoso B, Sar C, Gamo Y, Kobayashi T, Arai I and Takahashi J. Effects of including β1-4

galacto-oligosaccharides, lactic acid bacteria or yeast culture on methanogenesis as well as energy and nitrogen metabolism in sheep. Anim. Feed Sci. Technol. 2004: 115: 313-326. https://doi.org/10.1016/j.anifeedsci.2004.03.007

[42] Mitsumori M and Sun W. Control of rumen microbial fermentation for mitigating methane emissions from the rumen. Asian-Aust. J. Anim. Sci. 2008: 21:144-154. http://www.ajas.info/

[43] Wilkie, A. C. Anaerob Digestion: Holistic vioprocessing of animal manures. in proceeding of the animal residuals management coference. Virginia. 2002. 1-12.

[44] Fernando WMADB, Ian JM, Goozee KG, Charles SB, Jayasena V and Martins RN. The role of dietary coconut for the prevention and treatment of Alzaimer's disease: potential mecanishm of action. Cambridge university press. 2015: 114 (1): 1 – 14. Doi: https://doi.org/10.1017/S0007114515001452[Opens in a new window]

[45] Odle Jack. New Insights into the utlilization of medium chain triglycherides by the neonate: observation from a piglet model. The Journal of nutrition. 1997: 127:1061-1067. https://doi.org/10.1093/jn/127.6.1061

[46] Fife, Bruce. The Healing Miracles of Coconut Oil, 3rd Edition. Piccadilly Books Ltd. 2003. http://www.coconut-oil.com.

[47] Andrea A, Papamandjaris, Diane, MacDougal E and Petter, JHJ. Medium chain fatty acid metabolism and energy expenditure: obesity treatment implications. Life science. 1998: 62 (14): 1203 - 1215.32. https://doi.org/10.1016/S0024-3205(97)01143-0

[48] Waghorn G. Beneficial and detrimental effects of diertary condenses tannins for suitable sheep and goat production-progress and challenges. Anim. Feed Sci. Technol. 2008: 147: 116 – 139. https://doi.org/10.1016/j.anifeedsci.2007.09.013

[49] Staerfl SM, Zeitz JO, Kreuzer M and Soliva CR. Methane conversion rate of bulls fattened on grass or maize silage as compared with the IPCC default values, and the long-term methane mitigation efficiency of adding acacia tannin, garlic, maca and lupine. Agriculture, Ecosystems and Environment. 2012: 148: 111-120. DOI: 10.1016/j.agee.2011.11.003

[50] Ningrat RWS, Zain M, Erpomen and Suryani, H. Effect of doses and different sources of tannis on in vitro ruminal methane, volatile fatty acid production and on bacteria and protozoa population. Asian J. of Anim. and Vet. Adv. 2017: 11 (5): 314-318. DOI: 10.3923/ajas.2017.47.53

[51] Zain M, Putri EM, Ningrat RWS, Erpomen, Makmur M. Effects of Supplementing *Gliricidia Sepium* on ration based ammoniated rice straw in ruminant feed to decrease methane gas production and to improve nutrient digestibility (in-vitro). Int. J. on Adv.Sci. Eng.In.Tech. 2020: 10:2. DOI:10.18517/ijaseit.10.2.11242

[52] Molina-Botero IC, Arroyave-Jaramilloa J, Valencia-Salazarb S, Barahona-Rosalesc R, Aguilar-Péreza CF, Burgosa AA, Arangod J, Ku-Veraa JC. Effects of tannins and saponins contained in foliage of *Gliricidia sepium* and pods of *Enterolobium cyclocarpum* on fermentation, methane emissions and rumen microbial population in crossbred heifers. Animal Feed and Science Technology. 2019: 251. https://doi.org/10.1016/j.anifeedsci.2019.01.011

[53] Yang K, Wei C, Zhao GY, et al. Effects of dietary supplementing tannic acid in the ration of beef cattle on rumen fermentation, methane emission,

microbial flora and nutrient digestibility. J Anim Physiol Anim Nutr (Berl). 2017: 101: 302-10. DOI: 10.1111/jpn.12531

[54] Tan HY, Sieo CC, Abdullah N, Liang JB, Huang XD, et al. Effects of condensed tannins from Leucaena on methane production, rumen fermentation and populations of methanogens and protozoa in vitro. Anim Feed Sci Technol. 2011. 169: 185-193. https://doi.org/10.1016/j.anifeedsci.2011.07.004

[55] Patra AK, and Saxena J. Dietary phytochemicals as rumen modi ers: a review of the e ects on microbial populations. Antonie van Leeuwenhoek. 2009: 96: 363-375.

[56] Wina E, Muetzel S and Becker K. The dynamics of major brolytic microbes and enzyme activity in the rumen in response to short- and long-term feeding of Sapindus rarak saponins. Journal of Applied Microbiology. 2006b: 100 (1), 114-122. https://doi.org/10.1111/j.1365-2672.2005.02746.x

[57] Miah MY, Rahman MS, Islam MK and Monir MM. Effects of saponin and L-carnitine on the performance and reproductive fitness of male broiler. Int J Poult Sci. 2004: 3: 530 – 533.

[58] Anantasook N, Wanapat M, Gunun P, and Cherdthong A. Reducing methane production by supplementation of Terminalia chebula RETZ. containing tannins and saponins. Animal Science Journal. 2016: 87: 783-790. https://doi.org/10.1111/asj.12494

[59] Gerlach K, Pries M, Tholen E, Schmithausen AJ, Buscher W, Sudekum KH. Effect of condensed tannins in rations of lactating dairy cows on production variables and nitrogen use efficiency. J. Anim. 2018: 14 (9): 1847 -1855. https://doi.org/10.1017/S1751731117003639

[60] Arowolo MA and He J. Use of probiotics and botanical extracts to improve ruminant production in the tropics: A review. Animal Nutrition. 2018: 4: 241-249. https://doi.org/10.1016/j.aninu.2018.04.010

[61] Ningrat RWS, Zain M, Elihasridas, Makmur M, Putri M, Sari YC. Effect of dietary supplementation based on ammoniated palm frond with saccharomyces cerevisiae and gambir leaves waste on nutrient intake and digestibility, daily gain and methane production of simental cattle. Adv. In Anim.and Vet. Sci. 2020: 8(12): 1325-1332. http://dx.doi.org/10.17582/journal.aavs/2020/8.12.1325.1332

[62] Carrula JE, Kreuzer M, Machmiller A, Hess HD. Supplementation of *Acacia mearnsii* tannins decreases methanogenesis and urinary nitrogen in forage-fed sheep. Aust. J. Agric. Res. 2005: 56:961-970. https://doi.org/10.1071/ AR05022

[63] Goel G, Makkar HPS, Becker K. Effects of *Sesbania sesban* and *Carduus pycnocephalus* leaves and Fenugreek (*Trigonella foenum-graecum* L.) seeds and their extracts on partitioning of nutrients from roughage- and concentrate- based feeds to methane. Anim. Feed Sci. Technol. 2008: 147: 72- 89. https://doi.org/10.1016/j.anifeedsci.2007.09.010

[64] Piñeiro-Vázquez A, Canul-Solis J, Jiménez-Ferrer G, Alayón- Gamboa J, Chay-Canul A, Ayala-Burgos A, Aguilar-Pérez C, Ku-Vera J. Effect of condensed tannins from Leucaena leucocephala on rumen fermentation, methane production and population of rumen protozoa in heifers fed low-quality forage. Asian-Australas J. Anim. Sci. 2018: 31:1738- 1746. https://doi.org/10.5713/ajas.17.0192

Chapter 7

Nutritional Interventions to Reduce Methane Emissions in Ruminants

Lipismita Samal and Susanta Kumar Dash

Abstract

Methane is the single largest source of anthropogenic greenhouse gases produced in ruminants. As global warming is a main concern, the interest in mitigation strategies for ruminant derived methane has strongly increased over the last years. Methane is a natural by-product of anaerobic microbial (bacteria, archaea, protozoa, and fungi) fermentation of carbohydrates and, to a lesser extent, amino acids in the rumen. This gaseous compound is the most prominent hydrogen sink product synthesized in the rumen. It is formed by the archaea, the so-called methanogens, which utilize excessive ruminal hydrogen. Different nutritional strategies to reduce methane production in ruminants have been investigated such as dietary manipulations, plant extracts, lipids and lipid by-products, plant secondary metabolites, flavonoids, phenolic acid, statins, prebiotics, probiotics, etc. With the range of technical options suggested above, it is possible to develop best nutritional strategies to reduce the ill effects of livestock on global warming. These nutritional strategies seem to be the most developed means in mitigating methane from enteric fermentation in ruminants and some are ready to be applied in the field at the moment.

Keywords: methane, rumen fermentation, greenhouse gases, climate change, mitigation strategies

1. Introduction

Methane is the single largest source of anthropogenic greenhouse gases (GHG) produced in agricultural systems, especially in ruminant husbandry. It is estimated that 18% of the annual GHG emissions come from different types of livestock and that 37% of methane (CH_4) comes from fermentation processes in ruminants. As global warming is a main concern, the interest in mitigation strategies for ruminant derived methane is strongly increased over the last years. Enteric methane (~87%) is produced in rumen, the remaining 13% being released from fermentation in the large intestine [1]. Methane is a natural by-product of microbial fermentation of carbohydrates and, to a lesser extent, amino acids in the rumen. In rumen, the diverse and dense microbial populations consisting of protozoa, fungi and bacteria act on feed particles to degrade plant polysaccharides and produce volatile fatty acids (VFAs; mainly acetate, propionate and butyrate) and gases (CO_2 and H_2) as main end products. Methanogens use the excess of H_2 from NADH (reduced form of nicotinamide adenine dinucleotide) and CO_2 as the principal substrates to produce CH_4. About 82% of the CH_4 formed comes from H_2 reduction of CO_2, while about 18% is derived from formate. However, two genera of methanogens: the Methanosarcina and Methanosaeta can convert acetate to CO_2 and CH_4 (acetoclastic methanogenesis) [2]. Since methane contains energy, its emission during rumen fermentation is considered to be a loss of feed energy that is equivalent to 2–12% of dietary gross energy of animal feed.

2. Greenhouse gas effect

Since last few decades, the increased emission of GHG in the atmosphere has drawn worldwide attention due to global warming and stratospheric ozone depletion. The absorption and emission of infrared radiation by these atmospheric gases warm earth's surface and lower atmosphere. It ultimately leads to increased air, land and ocean temperatures and which in turn can increase annual precipitation in high rainfall regions and decrease precipitation in regions of low rainfall [3]. Global warming is the increase in average temperature of the earth's near-surface air and ocean since the mid-twentieth century and its projected continuation. In the twentieth century, average atmospheric temperature near the surface of the earth rose by 0.6 ± 0.2°C from 14°C. It is estimated that global temperature would increase by 1.4–5.8°C between 1990 and 2100. The Intergovernmental Panel on Climate Change (IPCC) concludes that most of the temperature increases since the mid-twentieth century is 'very likely' due to the increase in anthropogenic GHG concentrations.

The IPCC included six gases as GHG viz. CO_2, CH_4, nitrous oxide (N_2O), hydroflurocarbons, perflurocarbons and sulfur hexafluoride (SF_6). The first three gases in the atmosphere are produced as a result of agricultural and livestock activities. While CO_2 represents 73.5% of the total GHG, CH_4, N_2O and others represent 16.8%, 8.7% and 0.7% respectively. Since 1950, atmospheric CO_2 has increased 28%, while CH_4 has increased 70%. Methane, over the first 20 years after release, has 80-times more warming potential as a GHG than CO_2 [4]. Methane is also considered a highly potent GHG because of its ability to trap infrared radiation 20 times more effectively than CO_2 [5]. The warming potential of CO_2, CH_4 and N_2O is 1, 23 and 298, respectively. However, the life span of CH_4 in the atmosphere is 12 years while those of CO_2 and N_2O is 100 and 120 years respectively.

3. Livestock role in climate change

India possesses about one fifth of the world's total livestock population, which is being held responsible for the large contribution to the GHG emission. The livestock industry contributes ~18% of global GHG emissions. It accounts for 35% of CH_4, 9% of CO_2 and 65% of human-related N_2O emissions [6]. Enteric fermentation [7] and storage of slurry [6] are the main sources of anthropogenic CH_4 emissions. The output of methane emitted from ruminants accounts for one fifth of that in atmosphere. Methane emissions from ruminant livestock (cattle, buffalo, sheep and goat) were estimated at ~2.2 billion tonnes of CO_2 equivalent, accounting for ~80% of agricultural CH_4 and 37% of the total anthropogenic CH_4 emissions [8].

4. Rumen fermentation and methanogenesis

Digestion of feed in the rumen is the result of anaerobic fermentation involving various groups of microbes (bacteria, archaea, protozoa, and fungi). Methane is formed by the archaea, the so-called methanogens, which utilize excessive ruminal H_2. The activity of H_2-utilizing methanogenic archaea in rumen reduces the end product inhibition of H_2, thereby allowing more rapid fermentation of feed. Methane keeps the partial pressure of H_2 in the rumen contents very low, promoting the regeneration of reduced pyridine nucleotides by H_2 gas formation through hydrogenase activity instead of formation of lactate and ethanol by alcohol- or lactate-dehydrogenases. Even a small amount of H_2 in rumen can limit the oxidation of sugar, VFAs conversion and hydrogenase activity, if alternative pathways for disposal are absent [9].

The major factors influencing CH_4 emissions from ruminants are: (a) level of feed intake, (b) type of carbohydrates fed and (c) alteration of the ruminal microflora. When CH_4 reduction is attempted, it is therefore necessary to consider alternative hydrogen sinks to methanogenesis. Methanogenesis is the primary pathway followed by propionate production (fumarate reduction). Thus, a strategy for methane mitigation should be developed concomitantly with a strategy to enhance propionate production.

5. Nutritional interventions to reduce enteric methane emission

Nutritional strategies seem to be the most developed means in mitigating CH_4 from enteric fermentation in ruminants. Modes of action could be direct effects on methanogens [by medium-chain fatty acids (MCFA)], anti-protozoal effects [by saponins, MCFA and polyunsaturated fatty acids (PUFA)] or inhibiting organic matter (especially fiber) digestion followed by a lower H_2 supply to the methanogens [by condensed tannins (CT), MCFA, PUFA].

5.1 Manipulating nutrient composition of the diet

The feed quality and feed digestibility are the major determinants of energy available for animal growth and, therefore, of the performance of ruminants and of CH_4 production. Types and dietary proportions of carbohydrates are largely affecting ruminal fermentation conditions (especially pH), VFA profile and, concomitantly, CH_4 formation. The efficiency of nutrient utilization by microbial organisms in the rumen controls the fermentation process, which in turn affects the activity of methanogens relative to other microbial species. The forage-based diets result in generally higher enteric CH_4 formation than concentrates (grain-based feeds) in the diet. Dairy cows emitted less enteric CH_4 when fed a corn-based diet compared to ryegrass hay [10].

Starch, the main component of concentrate-rich diets, is mostly degradable to propionate which is a competitive H_2 sink to methanogenesis. In contrast, concentrates rich in sugars might have a higher methanogenic potential than starch or even fiber in dairy cows [11, 12], but this presumably only when a high ruminal pH is maintained [13]. An in vitro study [13] with starch and sucrose at different ruminal pH levels showed a higher CH_4 formation for sucrose, especially at high ruminal pH. This was mainly due to an increase in fiber digestion with the addition of sucrose. Diets containing feeds with elevated contents of distinct carbohydrates have gained attention in reducing CH_4 emissions. Grass cultivars selected for high contents of sugar (e.g., high-sugar ryegrass) might be an option for enteric CH_4 mitigation. However, grass-based feeding systems compared to those including maize silage have been reported to result in higher CH_4 emissions per unit of animal product [13]. Dohme-Meier et al. [14] observed that even feeding hay with a medium water-soluble carbohydrate (WSC) content (16%) can lead to a ruminal pH of <6 to which the methanogens are susceptible. When the ruminal pH is unaltered by feeding different grasses, methanogenesis could be increased by extra WSC and then sugars exhibit a higher methanogenic potential than starch [15]. There will be higher methane emission when WSC replaces the rumen degradable protein instead of fiber [16].

Forage quality can be improved through feeding forages with lower fiber and higher soluble carbohydrates, changing from C4 tropical grasses to C3 temperate species, or grazing less mature pastures. These options can also reduce CH_4 production [13]. Methane production per unit of cellulose digested has been shown to be 3 times that of hemicellulose, while cellulose and hemicelluloses ferment at a slower rate than non-structural carbohydrate, thus yielding more CH_4 per unit of substrate digested [17]. Methane emissions are also commonly lower with higher proportions of forage legumes in the diet, partly due to lower fiber content, faster rate of passage and, in some cases, the presence of condensed tannins [13].

5.2 Supplementation of lipids and lipid by-products

5.2.1 Dietary lipids

The use of lipids is considered as one of the promising dietary alternatives to depress ruminal methanogenesis. The effectiveness of fat supplementation depends mainly on the fat source, fatty acid profile, form of fat and the amount of supplemented fat [13]. Possible mechanisms by which added lipid can reduce enteric methane production include: (a) by reduction of fiber digestion (mainly in long-chain fatty acids); (b) by lowering of dry matter intake (if total dietary fat exceeds 6–7%); (c) by decreasing organic matter fermentation (d) through direct inhibition of activities of different microbes including methanogens and hydrogen producing microorganisms; (e) through suppression of rumen protozoa; and (f) to a limited extent through biohydrogenation of unsaturated fatty acids which serve as a hydrogen sink, although only 1–2% of the metabolic hydrogen in the rumen is used for this purpose [13, 17]. Fat can reduce CH_4 emissions by 4–5% (g/kg DMI) for every 1% increase in the fat content of the diet. Addition of different vegetable oils (soybean, coconut, canola, rapeseed, sunflower, linseed etc.) to ruminant diets have been shown to reduce CH_4 production between 18% and 62% in Rusitec fermenters [18], sheep [19], beef cattle [20] and dairy cows [21]. Beauchemin et al. [13] estimated a reduction of enteric CH_4 formation of 0.56% per g of lipid supplied per kg diet DM. Plant oils rich in MCFA such as coconut oil [major component is lauric acid (C14:0)] are known to inhibit rumen methanogenesis [18]. The addition of coconut oil to forage and concentrate rations supplemented to Charolais steers showed a reduction in voluntary intake and protozoa population and this was reflected in low CH_4 emissions, without affecting livestock production [22]. The lauric acid (C14:0) is more potent in CH_4 reduction than palmitic (C16:0), stearic (C18:0) and linoleic (C18:2) fatty acids in a semicontinuous fermenter that simulates the rumen (RUSITEC) [18]. A similar reduction in CH_4 was observed in batch cultures, in which coconut oil and lauric acid were directly compared. It showed that lauric acid inhibited methanogenesis to a greater extent [23]. The ability of lauric acid to decrease cell viability of Methanobrevibacter ruminantium has been reported [24]. The lauric acid treatment, possibly through its effect on protozoa physically associated with archaea, resulted in an increase in the archaeal methanogenic genus Methanosphaera and a decrease in Methanobrevibacter [25]. Besides lauric acid, other MCFA such as myristic acid, or a combination of both and PUFA like linolenic acid and linoleic acid were shown to be effective, but might also negatively influence feed intake and digestibility. The vegetable and fish oils significantly decreased CH_4 production after 14 d but not after 11 weeks of feeding in dairy cows [26]. However, persistence of the mitigating effect of dietary oil was observed in the study of Martin et al. [27] with flaxseed in dairy cows. Meta-analyses by Moate et al. [28] documented a consistent decrease in CH_4 production with fat supplementation. Other studies have reported a 27% reduction in CH_4 emission with the supplementation of fish oil and sunflower oil 500 mg/d each when fed to dairy cows in short periods (14 days) [26]. The reduction in methanogesis with oils/lipids appears to be the result of inhibition of microbial flora especially protozoa.

5.2.2 Lipid by-products

High-oil by-products from the biofuel industries such as dry distillers grains (DDG), wet distillers grains (WDG), dry distillers grains with solubles (DDGS), wet distillers grains with solubles (WDGS) and mechanically extracted oilseed meals are natural anti-methanogenic unconventional feeds. There was decrease in methane emission up to 24% when barley was replaced by DDG thereby supplementing an additional 3% lipid to the dietary DM in beef cattle [29]. Hales et al. [30] fed diets containing 0 to 45% WDGS (substituting steam-flaked corn) to Jersey steers and observed a linear increase in CH_4 emission per unit of DMI (up to 64% increase with the highest inclusion rate). Another product of the biodiesel industry, glycerol, has been shown to promote CH_4 production during ruminal fermentation in vitro. The inclusion of glycerol as a major component of the diet has been reported in beef cattle [31, 32], and inclusions of 10–20% in diet DM have been used without negatively affecting lamb performance [33]. When included up to 21% of diet DM, glycerol did not affect nutrient digestibility or CH_4 emissions of lambs fed barley-based finishing diets [34].

5.3 Plant secondary metabolites

Plant secondary metabolites (PSM) are groups of chemical bioactive compounds [tannins, saponins, essential oils (EO), alkaloids, flavonoids, glucosides, amines, non-protein amino acids, organosulfur compounds] in plants that are not involved in the primary biochemical processes of growth and reproduction but are meant for protection of the host plant against invasion by the pathogenic microbes. This highly specific anti-microbial activity is being exploited to modulate the rumen microbial ecosystem to alter rumen fermentation thereby decreasing methane production.

5.3.1 Tannins

Tannins are plant polyphenols of varying molecular size and exist in two forms in plants: hydrolysable tannin (HT) and condensed tannin (CT). Tannins, as feed supplements or as tanniferous plants have shown potential for reducing CH_4 emission by up to 20% [35]. Different types of tannin containing forages decreased CH_4 emission in vitro. The CH_4 inhibiting potential of tannins might be due to a direct effect on ruminal methanogens and an indirect effect on lower feed degradation leading to a decreased hydrogen production. Tannins and phenolic monomers have been found to be toxic for some of the rumen microbes, especially ciliate protozoa, fiber degrading bacteria and methanogenic archaea, and as a result methanogenesis in the rumen can also be reduced. The anti-methanogenic effect of tannins depends on its dietary concentration and is positively related to the number of hydroxyl groups in their structure. The hydrolyzable tannins tend to act by directly inhibiting rumen methanogens whereas the effect of condensed tannins (CT) on CH_4 production is more through inhibition of fiber digestion. In many studies (in vitro and in vivo) it has been demonstrated that with temperate legumes (*Hedysarium coronarium*, *Lespedeza cuneata*, *Lotus corniculatus* and *Lotus uliginosus*) and tropical legumes (*Calliandra calothyrsus*, *Flemingia macrophylla*) that contain CT, it is possible to reduce methanogenesis. The methane suppression effect of CT containing legumes, such as *Lotus pedunculatus* or *Acacia mearnsii*, relative to forages without tannins has been shown in sheep [36], cows [37] and goats [38]. *Ficus bengalensis*, *Autocarous integrifolis* and *Azadirachta indica* had also been shown to reduce methane production [39]. Ramirez-Restrepo and Barry [36] indicated that the CT-rich legumes such as *L. corniculatus* and sulla (*Hedysarum coronarium*) showed reduced methane production relative to forages without tannins (*Chicorium intybus*). In goats fed with the CT containing forage Sericea lespedeza, Puchala et al. [40] observed a reduction in CH_4 loss of over 30%. Methanol extract of harad (*Terminalia chebula*) caused 95% reduction in CH_4 production in vitro at the level of 0.25 ml/30 ml incubation medium and complete inhibition was observed when the level of extract was double [41]. In goats consuming different levels of CT from *Lespedeza striata*, there was a reduction in the emission of CH_4, while in the same study feeding Sorghum bicolor with lower levels of CT showed no reduction of enteric production of CH_4 [38].

5.3.2 Saponins

Saponins are naturally occurring surface-active glycosides with foaming characteristics, present in many plant species, wild plants as well as, cultivated crops. They usually consist of a sugar moiety linked to a hydrophobic compound, either triterpenoid or steroid in nature. Saponins reduce CH_4 production via inhibition of either protozoa or methanogens or both. These inhibited protozoa at relatively low concentrations whereas higher concentrations were required to kill or suppress methanogenic archaea. McAllister and Newbold [9] have suggested that a decrease in methanogens associated with protozoa as exo- and endosymbionts could be the main mechanism by which saponin feeding reduces methanogenesis and methanogens associated with protozoa are estimated to be responsible for 9–37% of the total CH_4 production in the rumen. Anti-methanogenic activity of saponins is believed to occur by limiting hydrogen availability to methanogens and re-channeling of metabolic hydrogen from methane to propionate production in the rumen. In addition, saponins, due to their chemical structure, may display anti-bacterial properties by reducing the number of bacteria producing H_2 thus resulting in the inhibition of H_2 production thereby reducing CH_4 formation. Goel and Makkar [42] summarized that there was no difference in the CH_4 mitigation effect between steroidal saponins (*Yucca schidigera*) and triterpenoid saponins (*Quillaja saponaria*). Studies from China have reported decreased CH_4 in ruminants treated with tea triterpenoid saponins (TS) but also substantial changes in microbial populations, including a reduction in protozoal counts [43]. Therefore, a reduction in the rumen protozoa population as a result of inclusion of TS in the diet could result in a decrease in enteric CH_4 production. Zhou et al. [44] reported that addition of TS reduced CH_4 production mainly by inhibiting protozoa, increasing molar proportions of propionate and decreasing acetate/propionate ratio without adversely altering relative ruminal abundance of fungi and cellulolytic bacteria. According to Lila et al. [45], supplementation of feed rations consisting of meadow hay and concentrate with saponins reduces CH_4 production in steers by 12.7%, while in the in vitro conditions during 24 h incubation, the reduction amounted ~15–44%. Hess et al. [46] reported that the daily CH_4 production was reduced by 6.5% due to supplementation of *Sapindus saponaria* fruits in sheep receiving tropical grass hay-concentrate diet.

Hess et al. [47] found that supplementation with *S. saponaria* saponin at 100 mg/g DM reduces methanogenesis by about 20% with no influence on the population of methanogens in the in vitro conditions. Wang et al. [48] reported a decreased CH_4 formation when feeding sarsaponins to sheep (0.13 g/kg diet). Saponins from *Sapindus murkossi* extracted with the use of ethanol, more effectively affect the process of methanogenesis in comparison to water and methanol extracts [49]. High effectiveness in the reduction of CH_4 production in the rumen ecosystem is possible to achieve also with the use of unextracted plant saponins, provided in the form of leaves or seeds (*Sesbana sesban*; *Trigonella foenum-graecum*). Seeds of temperate climate legumes (e.g., lupines, peas) are known to contain certain levels of tannins, and also of saponins.

5.3.3 Essential oils

Approximately 10–25% reduction of methane may be achievable through the addition of dietary oils in ruminants [13]. The CH_4 mitigating effect of essential oils might be due to suppression of methanogens. Another effect is the increase in the propionate-to-acetate ratio resulting in lower amounts of H_2 available. Plant breeding may in future offer opportunities to increase oil levels in selected forages and therefore increase oil intake directly as animals graze. Clear CH_4 mitigating effects were found in several in vitro studies when supplementing essential oils from garlic, thyme, oregano, cinnamon, rhubarb, frangula, etc. Garlic oil (principal component is diallyl disulfide), cinnamon oil (principal component is cinnamaldehyde), clove bud (principal component is eugenol), hot peppers (principal component is capsaicin) and anise oil may reduce methane production in the rumen by increasing the propionate-to-acetate ratio [50]. A study showed the potential anti-methanogenic properties of cashew nut shell liquid (active components are anacardic acid, cardanol and cardol), when added to batch cultures at the rate of 200 μg/ml of incubated volume [51]. A commercial blend of essential oils failed to decrease CH_4 production in vivo despite decreasing the digestibility of all nutrients [20]. The lack of response in vivo is partly attributed to the adaptation of microbes, but also to the use of lower doses compared to those in the in vitro experiments. The mustard seed oil and Japanese horseradish oil contain volatile compounds i.e. allyl isothiocyanate which has been reported to decrease CH_4 production in vitro. Use of peppermint oil (*Mentha piperita*) in low concentration of 1 or 2 μl/l, respectively resulted in linear reduction in methanogenesis (61%) together with the limitation on the number of methanogens (82%) and a decrease in the protozoan activity measured by ^{14}C-radio-isotopic technique [49]. Some researchers carried out a phylogenetic analysis of the rumen ecosystem and reported a tendency towards an increase in the diversity of methanogens in comparison to *Methanosphaera stadtmanae*, *M. smithii* and some uncultured groups with cinnamaldehyde, garlic and juniper berry oil supplementation [52]. When ajwain oil and lemon grass oil in 1: 1 ratio @ 0.05% of dry matter intake were fed to buffalo calves, methane production (L/kg digestible organic matter intake) was reduced by 16.7% [53] and feeding of these additives did not affect feed intake, rumen pH, or rumen metabolites [54].

5.3.4 Combination of different plant secondary metabolites

When EO-rich garlic and saponin-rich soapnut in 2:1 ratio @ 2% of DMI were fed to buffalo calves, methane production (L/kg digestible organic matter intake) was reduced by 12.9% [53] and feeding of these additives did not affect feed intake, rumen pH, or rumen metabolites except ammonia and enzyme profile [54].

When EO-rich garlic, saponin-rich soapnut, tannin-rich harad and EO-rich ajwain in 2:1:1:1 ratio@ 1% of DMI were fed to buffalo calves, methane production (L/kg digestible organic matter intake) was reduced by 8.4% [53] and feeding of these additives did not affect feed intake, rumen pH, or rumen metabolites except ammonia and enzyme profile [54].

5.4 Flavonoids

Oskoueian et al. [55] evaluated the effects of different flavonoids such as flavone, myricetin, naringin, catechin, rutin, quercetin, and kaempferol at the concentration of 4.5% of the substrate (dry matter basis) on the rumen microbial activity in vitro. These flavonoids suppressed CH_4 production significantly ($P < 0.05$). Total populations of protozoa and methanogens were significantly ($P < 0.05$) suppressed by naringin and quercetin. The researchers concluded that naringin and quercetin at the concentration of 4.5% of the substrate (dry matter basis) were potential metabolites to suppress CH_4 production without any negative effects on rumen microbial fermentation.

5.5 Phenolic acid

Caffeic acid (CA), a phenolic acid, serves as a promising rumen CH_4 inhibitor. It modulates methanogenesis and rumen fermentation mainly by affecting the growth of cellulolytic bacteria in vitro [56]. Kayembe et al. [57] reported the order of toxicity to methanogens by different phenolic monomers as follows: benzene > phenol > resorcinol > hydroquinone > pyrogallol which is attributed to the number of hydroxyl groups on the aromatic compound. Increase in the number of hydroxyl groups leads to decrease in toxicity to methanogens.

5.6 Statins

Fungal statins are used in human beings to reduce cholesterolemia. They inhibit 3-hydroxy-3-methylglutaryl coenzyme A (HMG-CoA) reductase which is a key enzyme in the cholesterol production pathway [58]. Unlike bacteria, archaea need HMG-CoA reductase for their membrane lipid synthesis. So, it has been hypothesized that statins can inhibit archaea by inhibiting HMG-CoA reductase [59, 60]. The effects of statins on methanogenesis and overall rumen fermentation vary depending on statin type and concentration. Hydrophobic statins, such as simvastatin and atorvastatin, seem to be more effective compared to the hydrophilic statins, such as rosuvastatin [61]. Several in vitro and in vivo studies have examined the potential of statins such as lovastatin and mevastatin to reduce rumen CH_4 production, but results were inconclusive [62, 63]. The concentrations of statins that decreased CH_4 production without negative effects on rumen fermentation spanned a wide range [64, 65].

5.7 Other metabolites

Methane inhibition has been demonstrated with dietary supplementation of various plant extracts, without identification of the active agents. Broudiscou et al. [66] investigated the effect of 13 plant extracts in continuous culture and showed that *Equisetum arvense* and *S. officinalis* had possible inhibitory effect on CH_4 production. Patra et al. [41] studied the effect of water, methanol and ethanol extracts of *Acacia concinna*, *T. chebula*, *T. bellirica*, *Emblica officinalis* and *A. indica* in vitro and observed reduction in CH_4 production by *T. chebula*.

A similar study [67] comparing *Y. schidigera* extract to *Castanea sativa* wood extract (containing HT and lignan) in in vitro rumen models showed effects on CH_4 production only at very high levels. Although rich in a long list of plant secondary metabolites, macahypocotyls and lupine seeds had no effect on enteric CH_4 formation [68]. Lupine seeds promoted methanogenesis in relation to the energy content of the diet as the increase per unit of SCFA shows when feeding about 200 g lupine seeds/kg DM to sheep [69].

European scientists screened 500 plant species for their ability to inhibit CH_4 production and selected 7 novel plants i.e. Italian plumeless thistle (*Carduus pycnocephalus*, 30% inhibition), the Chinese peony (*Paeonia lactiflora*, 8–53%), the European aspen (*Populus tremula*, 25%), the sweet cherry (*Prunus avium*, 20%), goat willow (*Salix caprea*, 30%), English oak (*Quercus pedunculata*, 25%) and Sikkim rhubarb (*Rheum nobile*, 25%). Carduus and Rheum species were evaluated in a RUSITEC analysis. On a high forage diet, 16 and 22% inhibition of methanogenesis was noted, while less inhibition (5 and 15% respectively, not significant) was observed on a high concentrate diet. Japanese researchers [70] reported that plant-derived liquid (PDL) and yeast-derived surfactant (YDS) induced >95% reduction in CH_4 production in batch cultures and >70% in RUSITEC analysis. The PDL contains anacardic acid, a salicylic acid derivative with an alkyl group that inhibits Gram-positive bacteria including bacilli and staphylococci. Anacardic acid was suggested to be a propionate enhancer. The YDS disrupts the cell walls of Gram-positive rumen bacteria. Hydrogen and formate producers viz. *Ruminococcus flavefaciens*, *Ruminococcus albus*, *Butyrivibrio fibrisolvens* and *Eubacterium ruminantium* were sensitive and propionate and succinate producers viz. *Selenomonas ruminantium*, *Megasphaera elsedenii* and *Succinivibrio dextrinosolvens* were tolerant to PDL and YDS. So, the rumen fermentation is shifted towards more propionate and less CH_4 production. Sheep that were fed a diet supplemented with PDL or YDS showed a fermentation pattern that was similar to that observed in RUSITEC and was accompanied by similar bacterial population shifts. Spanghero et al. [71] examined the chemical composition and rumen fermentability of grape seeds in vitro. Grape seeds are characterized by high levels of total phenols and total tannins [71] which might result in anti-methanogenic effects. Hop cones are feeds rich in specific plant secondary metabolites especially acids like humulones and lupulones. These acids are known to have anti-microbial effects [48]. Nevertheless, in vitro ruminal fermentation (e.g. increased gas production and VFA) was affected by hop addition [48]. In contrast, hop cones neither affected rumen fermentative activity nor incubation liquid ammonia nor CH_4 formation [72].

5.8 Prebiotics

In ruminants, prebiotics can be used along with nitrate and probiotics to reduce CH_4 production. They enhance propionate production by stimulating Selenomonas, Succinomonas and Megasphera sp. and decrease acetate production by inhibiting Ruminococcus and Butyrivibrio sp. [73]. Administration of galacto-oligosaccharides (GOS) decreased nitrite accumulation in rumen and plasma and nitrate-induced methemoglobin, while retaining low CH_4 production. 11% reduction in CH_4 emission (liters/day) in GOS supplemented diet compared to control diet has been reported [74]. Inclusion of GOS increased propionate production and decreased CH_4 formation [75].

5.9 Direct-fed microbials or probiotics

These are microbial feed additives that have been developed to improve animal productivity by directly influencing rumen fermentation. Several in vitro studies have demonstrated that probiotics can reduce CH_4 production [76]. Probiotics used in ruminant nutrition are yeast-based products (YP). Convincing animal data on YP for mitigating CH_4 production are lacking. Researchers also inoculated the rumen with fungi (*Candida kefyr*) and lactic acid bacteria (*Lactococcus lactis*) along with nitrate supplementation to control methanogenesis and prevent nitrite formation, but no consistent animal data have been reported [77].

5.9.1 Yeast culture

Yeast cultures (i.e., *Saccharomyces cerevisiae* and *Aspergillus oryzae*) reduce CH_4 production in three ways; (i) by reducing protozoa numbers, (ii) by increasing butyrate or propionate production and (iii) by stimulation of acetogens to compete with methanogens or to co-metabolize hydrogen, thereby decreasing CH_4 formation. However, the effects of probiotics may be diet-dependent. Carro et al. [78] observed reduction in CH_4 production and protozoa numbers when supplemented Rusitec fermenters with *S. cerevisiae* culture with a forage 50:concentrate 50 diet, but no effects were found with a forage 70:concentrate 30 diet. Lynch and Martin [79] reported 20% reduction in CH_4 production after 48 h of incubation with *S. cerevisiae* culture in an in vitro system. Frumholtz et al. [76] observed 50% decrease in CH_4 production when supplemented Rusitec fermenters with *A. oryzae* culture. Mwenya et al. [73] reported that sheep fed 70:30 forage:concentrate diet produced 10% less CH_4 when received daily 4 g of yeast culture. In contrast, Mathieu et al. [80] reported that *S. cerevisiae* and *A. oryzae* did not affect CH_4 production in sheep fed 44:66 forage:concentrate diet. However, results are inconsistent and further research is required to screen a large number of yeast strains to isolate those with significant CH_4 abatement potential.

5.9.2 Acetogens

Reductive acetogens are bacteria present in adult ruminants that reduce two moles of CO_2 to acetate by oxidation of H_2 in rumen unlike hydrogenotrophic methanogens, which utilize H_2 to reduce CO_2 to CH_4. So, acetogens are in direct competition with the methanogens. However, the affinity of the reductive acetogens for H_2 is 10–100 times lower than the hydrogenotrophic methanogens and the low partial pressure of H_2 in the rumen is not conducive for the acetogens to grow autotrophically [81]. So, while acetogens are present in the rumen, methanogens effectively outcompete them for hydrogen [9]. Acetogenic bacteria demonstrate higher population densities and an ability to be dominant under some conditions (e.g., in some macropods) [82]. Acetogenic bacteria are present in the rumen at population densities which may reach that of methanogens but despite their presence, reductive acetogenesis is extremely difficult to induce in the rumen. When methanogens are inhibited from the rumen by some means, they are capable of using this excess hydrogen to form acetate. Researchers are investigating these reactions with the aim of survival of acetogenic bacteria in the rumen and hence the displacement of methanogenic bacteria. An alternative approach would be to screen a range of acetogenic bacteria for their activity in rumen fluid and to introduce the acetogens into the rumen as a feed supplement. Lopez et al. [83] reported that *Eubacterium limosum* ATCC 8486 and Ser 5 increased acetate production and decreased H_2 formation when they were added to cultures of mixed ruminal microorganisms along with 2-bromoethanesulfonic acid (BES). In a rumen fistulated wether with continuous infusion of a 2-BES solution showed adaptation by methanogens after initial inhibition but use of cattle caecal contents, which contained acetogens, removed this adaptation effect [84]. Nollet et al. [81] reported that addition of Peptostreptococcus productus to BES-treated ruminal samples inhibited CH_4 production. On the basis of feed intake, VFAs, population density and hydrogen utilization pattern, it was suggested that reductive acetogenesis can sustain a functional rumen in the absence of methanogens [85].

5.9.3 Methane oxidizers

Methanotrophs or methane oxidizing bacteria are a unique group of methylotrophic bacteria. They require CH_4 as their carbon and energy source. So, they can be used as direct-fed microbial preparations. The oxidation reaction will compete with the CH_4 production and this reaction is a strictly anaerobic process [86]. Therefore, methane oxidizers from gut and non-gut sources could be screened for their activity in rumen.

5.9.4 Bacteriocins

Bacteriocins are narrow spectrum anti-bacterial proteinaceous polymeric substances and are produced by different Gram-positive and Gram-negative bacteria. They are under the control of plasmid. They compete with microbial species for niches within the rumen system. So, they could be effective in inhibiting methanogens and redirecting H_2 to other reductive bacteria like acetogens and propionate producers [9]. Some bacteriocins produced by lactic acid bacteria have been identified as an alternative group of anti-microbials for manipulation of the rumen microbial ecosystem [87]. The first described bacteriocin, nisin that is produced by *L. lactis* ssp. lactis, has a methane-mitigating ability that was observed in a monensin-supplemented in vitro culture (20% inhibition without a negative effect on VFA production) [88]. Although no mechanism was proposed to explain its effect on rumen bacteria, nisin potentiates propionate production and possibly shows selective activity against Gram-positive rumen bacteria. Nisin is active even at low pH, decreases the acetate to propionate ratio. It has been reported that 36% methanogenesis was reduced by using nisin [88]. A combination of nisin and nitrate, an alternative electron receptor, has been reported to reduce CH_4 emissions in sheep [89]. Alazzeh et al. [90] reported that the use of some strains of propionibacteria have the potential to lower CH_4 production from mixed rumen cultures and this reduction is not always associated with an increase in propionate production. Klieve and Hegarty [91] suggested that bacteriocins could be used to decrease ruminal CH_4 production in vivo. But rather than using bacteriocins of exogenous origin, it is advantageous to use bacteriocin of rumen origin. Bovicin HC5, the semi-purified bacteriocin produced by *Streptococcus bovis* HC5 from the rumen, has been reported to suppress CH_4 production by 50% in vitro [92], and even low concentration of bovicin HC5 (128 activity units ml^{-1}) may be equally as useful as monensin in limiting CH_4 production in the rumen [92, 93]. The CH_4 content declined with pediocin, enterocin and combinations of both after 24 h incubation. Pediocin P1 and P2 decreased ($P < 0.05$) CH_4 level by 4.81% and 5.08%, respectively when compared to control and combinations of bacteriocin.

5.9.5 Fungal metabolites

Secondary fungal metabolites from Monascus spp. reduced enteric CH_4 emissions in sheep by 30%, decreased acetate to propionate ratio and reduced methanogen numbers in a short-term trial [65]. The red macroalgae or seaweed (*Asparagopsis taxiformis*) when added at 2% of substrate organic matter, decreased CH_4 emissions by 99% without reducing substrate digestibility or VFA production in laboratory rumen fermentation cultures [24]. *A. taxiformis* decreased enteric CH_4 production from sheep [94] and beef steers [95].

5.9.6 Methane reducing species

Mitsuokella jalaludinii has been demonstrated as an efficient CH_4 reducing agent in the rumen by competing with methanogens for hydrogen, necessary for growth by both [96]. *M. jalaludinii* decreases CH_4 production and improves rumen fermentation thereby improving feed efficiency in livestock.

5.10 Conclusion

Any sustainable solution to lower on-farm CH_4 emissions should be practical, cost-effective and have no substantial adverse effect on the profitability of ruminant livestock production. In this context, manipulating diet composition to induce changes in enteric fermentation characteristics remains the most feasible approach to lower CH_4 production. Therefore, efforts should be made to select feed ingredients and to identify forage plants containing secondary metabolites that can be used to inhibit methanogenesis selectively, but without adversely affecting feed utilization. Moreover, rumen is a dynamic ecosystem and rumen methanogenesis is a complex process. Since our understanding of rumen microbes is still incomplete, elucidation of microbial diversity and microbial interrelationships is absolutely essential for the successful manipulation of rumen fermentation towards a significant reduction in ruminant CH_4 emission.

Author details

Lipismita Samal* and Susanta Kumar Dash
Odisha University of Agriculture and Technology, Bhubaneswar, India

*Address all correspondence to: lipismitasamal@gmail.com

References

[1] Lascano CE, Cárdenas E. Alternatives for methane emission mitigation in livestock systems. Revista Brasileira de Zootecnia. 2010;**39**:175-182

[2] Deppenmeier U. The unique biochemistry of methanogenesis. Progress in Nucleic Acid Research and Molecular Biology. 2002;**71**:223-283

[3] Gerstengarbe FW, Werner P. Climate development in the last century-global regional. International Journal of Medical Microbiology. 2008;**298**:5-11

[4] Black JL, Davison TM, Box I. Methane emissions from ruminants in Australia: Mitigation potential and applicability of mitigation strategies. Animals. 2021;**11**:951

[5] Mohammed N, Ajisaka N, Lila Z, Hara K, Mikuni K, Hara K, et al. Effect of Japanese horseradish oil on methane production and ruminal fermentation in vitro and in steers. Journal of Animal Science. 2004;**82**:1839-1846

[6] Sejian V, Samal L, Bagath M, Suganthi RU, Lal R. Manure management: Gaseous emissions. In: Lal R, editor. Encyclopedia of Soil Science. 3rd ed. New York, USA: Taylor and Francis Publisher; 2017. pp. 1400-1405

[7] Chang J, Peng S, Ciais P, et al. Revisiting enteric methane emissions from domestic ruminants and their $\delta^{13}C_{CH4}$ source signature. Nature Communications. 2019;**10**:3420

[8] Patra AK, Yu Z. Effects of essential oils on methane production, fermentation, abundance and diversity of rumen microbial populations. Applied and Environmental Microbiology. 2012;**78**:4271-4280

[9] McAllister TA, Newbold CJ. Redirecting rumen fermentation to reduce methanogenesis. Australian Journal of Experimental Agriculture. 2008;**48**:7-13

[10] Klevenhusen F, Bernasconi SM, Kreuzer M, Soliva CR. Experimental validation of the Intergovernmental Panel on Climate Change default values for ruminant-derived methane and its carbon-isotope signature. Animal Production Science. 2010;**50**:159-167

[11] Hindrichsen IK, Wettstein HR, Machmuller A, Jörg B, Kreuzer M. Effect of the carbohydrate composition of feed concentrates on methane emission from dairy cows and their slurry. Environmental Monitoring and Assessment. 2005;**107**:329-350

[12] Ellis JL, Dijkstra J, Bannink A, Kebreab E, Hook SE, Archibeque S, et al. Quantifying the effect of monensin dose on the rumen volatile fatty acid profile in high-grain fed beef cattle. Journal of Animal Science. 2012;**90**:2717-2726

[13] Beauchemin KA, Kreuzer M, O'Mara F, McAllister TA. Nutritional management for enteric methane abatement: A review. Australian Journal of Experimental Agriculture. 2008;**48**:21-27

[14] Dohme-Meier F, Brand D, Arrigo Y, Münger A. Varrierende Gehalte an löslichen Kohlenhydraten im Wiesenfutter und ihr Einfluss auf die Pansenfermentation. In: Kreuzer M, Lanzini T, Wanner M, Bruckmaier R, Guidon D, editors. ETH Schriftenreihe zur Tierernährung. Vol. 34. Switzerland: ETH Zurich; 2011. pp. 69-73

[15] Hindrichsen IK, Kreuzer M. High methanogenic potential of sucrose compared with starch at high ruminal pH. Journal of Animal Physiology and Animal Nutrition. 2009;**93**:61-65

[16] Bannink A, Smits MCJ, Kebreab E, Mills JAN, Ellis JL, Klop A, et al. Simulating the effect of grassland management and grass ensiling on methane emission from lactating cows. The Journal of Agricultural Science. 2010;**148**:55-72

[17] Eckard RJ, Grainger C, De Klein CAM. Options for the abatement of methane and nitrous oxide from ruminant production—A review. Livestock Science. 2010;**130**:47-56

[18] Dohme F, Machmüller A, Wasserfallen A, Kreuzer M. Comparative efficiency of various fats rich in medium-chain fatty acids to suppress ruminal methanogenesis as measured with RUSITEC. Canadian Journal of Animal Science. 2000; **80**:473-484

[19] Ding X, Long R, Zhang Q, Huang X, Guo X, Mi J. Reducing methane emissions and the methanogen population in the rumen of Tibetan sheep by dietary supplementation with coconut oil. Tropical Animal Health and Production. 2012;**44**:1541-1545

[20] Beauchemin KA, McGinn SM. Methane emissions from beef cattle: Effects of fumaric acid, essential oil, and canola oil. Journal of Animal Science. 2006;**84**:1489-1149

[21] Brask M, Lund P, Weisbjerg MR, Hellwing AL, Poulsen M, Larsen MK, et al. Methane production and digestion of different physical forms of rapeseed as fat supplement in dairy cows. Journal of Dairy Science. 2013;**96**:2356-2365

[22] Lovett D, Lovell S, Stack L, Callan J, Finlay M. Effect of forage/concentrate ratio and dietary coconut oil level on methane output and performance of finishing beef heifers. Livestock Production Science. 2003;**84**:135-146

[23] Yabuuchi Y, Tani M, Matsushita Y, Otsuka H, Kobayashi Y. Effects of lauric acid on physical, chemical and microbial characteristics in the rumen of steers on a high grain diet. Animal Science Journal. 2007;**78**:387-394

[24] Zhou X, Meile L, Kreuzer M, Zeitz JO. The effect of lauric acid on methane production and cell viability of *Methanobrevibacter ruminantium*. Advances in Animal Biosciences. 2013;**4**(2):458

[25] Hristov AN, Callaway TR, Lee C, Dowd SE. Rumen bacterial, archaeal, and fungal diversity of dairy cows in response to ingestion of lauric or myristic acid. Journal of Animal Science. 2012;**90**:4449-4457

[26] Woodward SL, Waghorn GC, Thomson NA. Supplementing dairy cows with oils to improve performance and reduce methane—Does it work? Proceedings of the New Zealand Society of Animal Production. 2006;**66**:176-181

[27] Martin C, Pomiès D, Ferlay A, Rochette Y, Martin B, Chilliard Y, et al. Methane output and rumen microbiota in dairy cows in response to longterm supplementation with linseed or rapeseed of grass silage- or pasturebased diets. Proceedings of the New Zealand Society of Animal Production. 2011; **71**:242-247

[28] Moate PJ, Williams SRO, Grainger C, Hannah MC, Ponnampalam EN, Eckard RJ. Influence of cold-pressed canola, brewers grains and hominy meal as dietary supplements suitable for reducing enteric methane emissions from lactating dairy cows. Animal Feed Science and Technology. 2011; **166-167**:254-264

[29] McGinn SM, Chung YH, Beauchemin KA, Iwaasa AD, Grainger C. Use of corn distillers' dried grains to reduce enteric methane loss from beef cattle. Canadian Journal of Animal Science. 2009;**89**:409-413

[30] Hales KE, Cole NA, MacDonald JC. Effects of increasing concentrations of wet distillers grains with soluble in steam-flaked corn-based diets on energy metabolism, carbon-nitrogen balance and methane emissions of cattle. Journal of Animal Science. 2013;**91**:819-828

[31] Mach N, Bach A, Devant M. Effects of crude glycerine supplementation on performance and meat quality of Holstein bulls fed high-concentrate diets. Journal of Animal Science. 2009;**87**:632-638

[32] Parsons GL, Shelor MK, Drouillard JS. Performance and carcass traits of finishing heifers fed crude glycerin. Journal of Animal Science. 2009;**87**:653-657

[33] Gunn PJ, Neary MK, Lemenager RP, Lake SI. Effects of crude glycerine on performance and carcass characteristics of finishing wether lambs. Journal of Animal Science. 2010;**88**:1771-1776

[34] Avila-Stagno J, Chaves AV, He ML, Harstad OM, Beauchemin KA, McGinn SM, et al. Effects of increasing concentrations of glycerol in concentrate diets on nutrient digestibility, methane emissions, growth, fatty acid profiles, and carcass traits of lambs. Journal of Animal Science. 2013;**91**:829-837

[35] Staerfl SM, Amelchanka SL, Kälber T, Soliva CR, Kreuzer M, Zeitz JO. Effect of feeding dried high-sugar ryegrass ('AberMagic') on methane and urinary nitrogen emissions of primiparous cows. Livestock Science. 2012;**150**:293-301

[36] Ramirez-Restrepo CA, Barry TN. Alternative temperate forages containing compounds for improving sustainable productivity in grazing ruminants. Animal Feed Science and Technology. 2005;**120**:179-201

[37] Grainger C, Clarke T, Auldist MJ, Beauchemin KA, McGinn SM, Waghorn GC, et al. Potential use of Acacia mearnsii condensed tannins to reduce methane emissions and nitrogen excretion from grazing dairy cows. Canadian Journal of Animal Science. 2009;**89**:241-251

[38] Animut G, Goetsch AL, Puchala R, Patra AK, Sahlu T, Varel VH, et al. Methane emission by goats consuming different sources of condensed tannins. Animal Feed Science and Technology. 2008;**144**:228-241

[39] Bhatt VD, Dande SS, Patil NV, Joshi CG. Molecular analysis of the bacterial microbiome in the forestomach fluid from the dromedary camel (*Camelus dromedaries*). Molecular Biology Reports. 2013;**40**:3363-3371

[40] Puchala R, Min BR, Goetsch AL, Sahlu T. The effect of a condensed tannin-containing forage on methane emission by goats. Journal of Animal Science. 2005;**83**:182-186

[41] Patra AK, Kamra DN, Agarwal N. Effect of plant extracts on in vitro methanogenesis enzyme activities and fermentation of feed in the rumen liquor of buffalo. Animal Feed Science and Technology. 2006;**128**:276-291

[42] Goel G, Makkar HPS. Methane mitigation from ruminants using tannins and saponins. Tropical Animal Health and Production. 2012;**44**:729-739

[43] Wang JK, Ye JA, Liu JX. Effects of tea saponins on rumen microbiota, rumen fermentation, methane production and growth performance—A review. Tropical Animal Health and Production. 2012;**44**:697-706

[44] Zhou M, Chung YH, Beauchemin KA, Holtshausen L, Oba M, McAllister TA, et al. Relationship between rumen methanogens and methane production in dairy cows fed diets supplemented with a feed enzyme

additive. Journal of Applied Microbiology. 2011;**111**:1148-1158

[45] Lila ZA, Mohammed N, Kanda S, Kurihara M, Itabashi H. Sarsaponin effects on ruminal fermentation and microbes, methane production, digestibility and blood metabolites in steers. Asian-Australasian Journal of Animal Sciences. 2005;**12**:1746 (Abstr.)

[46] Hess HD, Beuret RA, Lotscher M, Hindrichsen KI, Machműller A, Carulla JE, et al. Ruminal fermentation, methanogensis and nitrogen utilization of sheep receiving tropical grass hay-concentrate diet offered with *Sapindus saponaria* fruits and Cratylia argentea foliage. Animal Science. 2004; **79**:177-189

[47] Hess HD, Kreuzer M, Diaz TE, Lascano CE, Carulla JE, Soliva CR, et al. Saponin rich tropical fruits affect fermentation and methanogenesis in faunated and defaunated rumen fluid. Animal Feed Science and Technology. 2003;**109**:79-94

[48] Wang Y, Chaves AV, Rigby FL, He ML, McAllister TA. Effects of hops on ruminal fermentation, growth, carcass traits and shedding of Escherichia coli of feedlot cattle. Livestock Science. 2010;**129**:135-140

[49] Agarwal N, Shekhar C, Kumar R, Chaudhary LC, Kamra DN. Effect of peppermint (*Mentha piperita*) oil on in vitro methanogenesis and fermentation of feed with buffalo rumen liquor. Animal Feed Science and Technology. 2009;**148**:321-327

[50] Calsamiglia S, Busquet M, Cardozo PW, Castillejos L, Ferret A. Invited review: Essential oils as modifiers of rumen microbial fermentation. Journal of Dairy Science. 2007;**90**:2580-2595

[51] Watanabe Y, Suzuki R, Koike S, Nagashima K, Mochizuki M, Forster RJ, et al. In vitro evaluation of cashew nut shell liquid as a methane inhibiting and propionate-enhancing agent for ruminants. Journal of Dairy Science. 2010;**93**:5258-5267

[52] Ohene-Adjei S, Chaves AV, McAllister TA, Benchaar C, Teather RM, Forster RJ. Evidence of increased diversity of methanogenic archaea with plant extract supplementation. Microbial Ecology. 2008;**56**:234-242

[53] Samal L, Chaudhary LC, Agarwal N, Kamra DN. Impact of phytogenic feed additives on growth performance, nutrient digestion and methanogenesis in growing buffaloes. Animal Production Science. 2016;**58**(6): 1056-1063

[54] Samal L, Chaudhary LC, Agarwal N, Kamra DN. Effect of plants containing secondary metabolites as feed additives on rumen metabolites and methanogen diversity of buffaloes. Animal Production Science. 2016; **56**:472-481

[55] Oskoueian E, Abdullah N, Oskoueian A. Effects of flavonoids on rumen fermentation activity, methane production, and microbial population. BioMed Research International. 2013; Article ID 349129, p. 8

[56] Jin Q, You W, Tan X, Liu G, Zhang X, Liu X, et al. Caffeic acid modulates methane production and rumen fermentation in an opposite way with high-forage or high-concentrate substrate in vitro. Journal of the Science of Food and Agriculture. 2021; **101**(7):3013-3020

[57] Kayembe K, Basosila L, Mpiana PT, Sikulisimwa PC, Mbuyu K. Inhibitory effects of phenolic monomers on methanogenesis in anaerobic digestion. British Microbiology Research Journal. 2013;**3**(1):32-41

[58] Sirtori CR. The pharmacology of statins. Pharmacological Research. 2014;**88**:3-11

[59] Wolin MJ, Miller TL. Control of rumen methanogenesis by inhibiting the growth and activity of methanogens with hydroxymethylglutaryl-SCoA inhibitors. International Congress Series. 2006;**1293**:131-137

[60] Gottlieb K, Wacher V, Sliman J, Pimentel M. Inhibition of methanogenic archaea by statins as a targeted management strategy for constipation and related disorders. Alimentary Pharmacology & Therapeutics. 2016;**43**:197-212

[61] Joch M, Vadroňová M, Výborná A, Jochová K. Inhibition of in vitro rumen methane production by three statins. Annals of Animal Science. 17th March, 2021. DOI: 10.2478/aoas-2021-0022

[62] Patra A, Park T, Kim M, Yu Z. Rumen methanogens and mitigation of methane emission by anti-methanogenic compounds and substances. Journal of Animal Science and Biotechnology. 2017;**8**:13

[63] Henderson G, Cook GM, Ronimus RS. Enzyme- and gene-based approaches for developing methanogen-specific compounds to control ruminant methane emissions: A review. Animal Production Science. 2018;**58**:1017-1026

[64] Soliva CR, Amelchanka SL, Duval SM, Kreuzer M. Ruminal methane inhibition potential of various pure compounds in comparison with garlic oil as determined with a rumen simulation technique (Rusitec). The British Journal of Nutrition. 2011; **106**:114-122

[65] Morgavi DP, Martin C, Boudra H. Fungal secondary metabolites from Monascus spp. reduce rumen methane production in vitro and in vivo. Journal of Animal Science. 2013;**91**:848-860

[66] Broudiscou LP, Papon Y, Broudiscou AF. Effects of dry plant extracts on fermentation and methanogenesis in continuous culture of rumen microbes. Animal Feed Science and Technology. 2000; **87**:263-277

[67] Sliwinski BJ, Soliva CR, Machmuller A, Kreuzer M. Efficacy of plant extracts rich in secondary constituents to modify rumen fermentation. Animal Feed Science and Technology. 2002;**101**:101-114

[68] Staerfl SM, Kreuzer M, Soliva CR. In vitro screening of unconventional feeds and various natural supplements for their ruminal methane mitigation potential when included in a maize-silage based diet. Journal of Animal and Feed Sciences. 2010;**19**:651-664

[69] Rémond D, Le Guen MP, Poncet C. Degradation in the rumen and nutritional value of lupin (*Lupinus albus* L.) seed proteins effect of extrusion. Animal Feed Science and Technology. 2003;**105**:55-70

[70] Kobayashi Y. Abatement of methane production from ruminants: Trends in the manipulation of rumen fermentation. Asian-Australasian Journal of Animal Sciences. 2010;**23**(3):410-416

[71] Spanghero M, Salem AZM, Robinson PH. Chemical composition, including secondary metabolites, and rumen fermentability of seeds and pulp of Californian (USA) and Italian grape pomaces. Animal Feed Science and Technology. 2009;**152**:243-255

[72] Stärfl SM. Influence of various forage-based feeding systems and supplementation strategies on enteric and slurry-derived methane emissions from fattening bulls and dairy cows [dissertation]. Germany: ETH Zurich for the degree of Doctor of Sciences; 2012. pp. 1-128

[73] Mwenya B, Santoso B, Sar C, Gamo Y, Kobayashi T, Arai I, et al. Effects of including β1-4 galacto-oligosaccharides lactic acid bacteria or yeast culture on methanogenesis as well as energy and nitrogen metabolism in sheep. Animal Feed Science and Technology. 2004;**115**:313-326

[74] Zhou X, Sar C, Kobayashi T, Takahashi J, Santoso B, Gamo Y, et al. Effects of probiotic vitacogen and ß1-4 galacto-oligosaccharides supplementation on methanogenesis and energy and nitrogen utilization in dairy cows. Asian-Australasian Journal of Animal Sciences. 2004;**17**(3): 349-354

[75] Santoso B, Mwenyaa B, Sara C, Gamoa Y, Kobayashia T, Morikawaa R, et al. Effects of supplementing galacto-oligosaccharides, *Yucca schidigera* or nisin on rumen methanogenesis, nitrogen and energy metabolism in sheep. Livestock Production Science. 2004;**91**:209-217

[76] Frumholtz P, Newbold C, Wallace R. Influence of *Aspergillus oryzae* fermentation extract on the fermentation of a basal ration in the rumen simulation technique (Rusitec). Journal of Agricultural Science. 1989;**113**:169-172

[77] Takahashi J. Some prophylactic options to mitigate methane emission from animal agriculture in Japan. Asian-Australasian Journal of Animal Sciences. 2011;**24**:285-294

[78] Carro MD, Lebzien P, Rohr K. Influence of yeast culture on the in vitro fermentation (Rusitec) of diets containing variable portions of concentrates. Animal Feed Science and Technology. 1992;**37**:209-220

[79] Lynch H, Martin S. Effects of *Saccharomyces cerevisiae* culture and Saccharomyces cerevisiae live cells on in vitro mixed ruminal microorganism fermentation. Journal of Dairy Science. 2002;**85**:2603-2608

[80] Mathieu F, Jouany JP, Senaud J, Bohatier J, Bertin G, Mercier M. The effect of Saccharomyces cerevisiae and *Aspergillus oryzae* on fermentations in the rumen of faunated and defaunated sheep; protozoal and probiotic interactions. Reproduction, Nutrition, Development. 1996;**36**:271-287

[81] Nollet L, Demeyer D, Verstraete W. Effect of 2-bromoethanesulfonic acid and Peptostreptococcus productus atcc 35244 addition on stimulation of reductive acetogenesis in the ruminal ecosystem by selective inhibition of methanogenesis. Applied and Environmental Microbiology. 1997;**63**(1):194-200

[82] Ouwerkerk D, Maguire AJ, McMillen L, Klieve AV. Hydrogen utilizing bacteria from the forestomach of eastern grey (*Macropus giganteus*) and red (*Macropus rufus*) kangaroos. Animal Production Science. 2009;**49**:1043-1051

[83] Lopez S, McIntosh FM, Wallace RJ, Newbold CJ. Effect of adding acetogenic bacteria on methane production by mixed rumen microorganisms. Animal Feed Science and Technology. 1999;**78**:1-9

[84] Immig I, Demeyer D, Fiedler D, Van Nevel C, Mbanzamihigo L. Attempts to induce reductive acetogenesis into a sheep rumen. Archiv für Tierernährung. 1996;**49**(4):363-370

[85] Fonty G, Joblin K, Chavarot M, Roux R, Naylor G, Michallon F. Establishment and development of ruminal hydrogenotrophs in methanogen-free lambs. Applied and Environmental Microbiology. 2007;**73**:6391-6403

[86] Hanson RS, Hanson TE. Methanotropic bacteria. Microbiological Reviews. 1996;**60**(2):439-471

[87] Chen H, Hoocver DG. Bacteriocins and their food applications. CRFSFS. 2003;**12**:82-99

[88] Callaway TR, Alexandra MS, De Melo C, Russell JB. The effect of nisin and monensin on ruminal fermentations in vitro. Current Microbiology. 1997; **35**:90-96

[89] Sar C, Mwenya B, Santoso B, Takaura K, Morikawa R, Isogai N, et al. Effect of *Escherichia coli* wild type or its derivative with high nitrite reductase activity on in vitro ruminal methanogenesis and nitrate/nitrite reduction. Journal of Animal Science. 2005;**83**:644-652

[90] Alazzeh AY, Sultana H, Beauchemin KA, Wang Y, Holo H, Harstad OM, et al. Using strains of Propionibacteria to mitigate methane emissions in vitro. Acta Agriculturae Scandinavica. 2012;**62**(4):263-272

[91] Klieve AV, Hegarty RS. Opportunities for biological control of ruminal methanogenesis. Australian Journal of Agricultural Research. 1999;**50**(8):1315-1320

[92] Lee SS, Hsu JT, Mantovani HC, Russell JB. The effect of bovicin HC5, a bacteriocin from *Streptococcus bovis* HC5, on ruminal methane production in vitro. FEMS Microbiology Letters. 2002;**217**:51-55

[93] Lima JR, Ribon AO, Russell JB, Mantovani HC. Bovicin HC5 inhibits wasteful amino acid degradation by mixed ruminal bacteria in vitro. FEMS Microbiology Letters. 2009;**292**:78-84

[94] Li X, Norman H, Kinley R, Laurence M, Wilmot M, Bender H, et al. Asparagopsis taxiformis decreases enteric methane production from sheep. Animal Production Science. 2016; **58**:681-688

[95] Roque BM, Venegas M, Kinley RD, de Nys R, Duarte TL, Yang X, et al. Red seaweed (*Asparagopsis taxiformis*) supplementation reduces enteric methane by over 80 percent in beef steers. PLoS One. 2021;**16**(3):e0247820

[96] Mamuad LL, Kim SH, Lee SS, Cho KK, Jeon CO, Lee SS. Characterization, metabolites and gas formation of fumarate reducing bacteria isolated from Korean Native Goat (*Capra hircus coreanae*). Journal of Microbiology. 2012;**50**:925-931

Chapter 8

Health Hazards of Toxic and Essential Heavy Metals from the Poultry Waste on Human and Aquatic Organisms

Adesakin Taiwo Adekanmi

Abstract

This research was conducted to examine the impact of some essential heavy metals used as a supplement during animal feed formulation and the toxic from unregulated discharges of untreated poultry waste into water bodies on man and aquatic organisms. During the processing of poultry feed, certain heavy metals are used as a supplement such as selenium, copper, zinc, iron etc. to enhance poultry meat and egg yield which is also increase the daily discharge of anthropogenic wastes into our environment that contain high concentration of heavy metals discharges into aquatic environment globally, especially in underdeveloped where this waste are not treated before discharge or used in agriculture as an organic fertilizer in planting crops as a result of this it become absorb by plants and could pose a serious health risk to man and aquatic species as well as affect the ecological balance that can be transfer to humans via the food chain. Some organisms are kills as a result of the toxic heavy metals in water and can affect their growths. Bio-accumulated in the body of certain species, such as fish, which are eaten by humans that causes devastating diseases such as Minamata and Itai-Itai. Regulation of the use some heavy metals as a supplement in feed production or complete removal of it in animal feed should be adopt in order to minimize the human health risks and environmental contamination associated with these animal waste.

Keywords: essential heavy metals, animals feed, health risk, supplement, growth, toxic metals

1. Introduction

Water covers about 70 per cent of the Earth's surface, makes up about 75 per cent of human body mass, and is the basic material that all living things need to live. The fact that water covers more than two-thirds of the Earth's surface makes it hard to believe that it is a scarce resource and that less than 1% of the total water on this planet is readily accessible for drinking or other uses. Approximately 97% of the earth's water is salt water contained in lakes or seas; just 3% is fresh water. However, 68 per cent of freshwater on Earth is enclosed in the Antarctic and Greenland ice caps (30%) while just 0.3 per cent is enclosed in surface waters, including lakes, rivers, reservoirs, springs and streams. Water quality can be defined by its physical, chemical, biological and esthetic characteristics (appearance and smell) as well as by its fitness for the beneficial uses it has in the past provided for human and animal drinking, for the promotion of a healthy aquatic life, for irrigation of the land and for recreation. A safe water ecosystem is when it meets the standard in term of water maintains a rich, diverse population of species and is conducive for the consumption of public health. Water is of course, the basic liquid medium for living matter; thus, it is uniquely vulnerable to contamination by living creatures, including those that cause disease to humans. Aquatic contamination occurs as a result of the introduction by humans of either direct discharges into the water body or indirect substances or/energy that may result in the degradation of the water quality of any water body that poses a danger to human health, harms living organisms and hinders aquatic activities such as fishing and polluted water quality with respect to its use. Contamination mechanisms including suspension, solution and biochemical alteration is not inherently separate and distinct from each other and all of these complex processes may only occur in water. However, growing anthropogenic activities, such as urbanization, Industries, agricultural waste, etc. and natural processes, reduce water quality and pose a danger to all modes of life. Most people live in underdeveloped countries still depend on unprotected/contaminated water sources as their primary sources of drinking water and at the same time, as their means of waste disposal, which can cause outbreaks of waterborne diseases. The discharge of industrial waste into water bodies constitutes approximately 62 per cent of the overall source of heavy metals such as lead (Pb), zinc (Zn), copper (Cu), nickel (Ni), cadmium (Cd) and chromium (Cr) [1]. It is important to write about contamination caused by heavy trace elements, since untreated waste materials discharged by industry or agriculture worldwide are very concerned about the current disposal of waste materials containing heavy metals such as mercury, cadmium, lead, copper and arsenic due to growing concentrations in many waters.

2. Poultry farm waste

Poultry farms are one of the world's leading sources of high-grade and palatable protein-rich food (eggs and meat) but domestic, industrial and agricultural poultry waste is regularly disposed of without treatment into water bodies, especially in most developing countries. Poultry farming is a lucrative global trade in animal husbandry that raises domesticated birds such as chickens, ducks, quails, pigeons, guinea fowl, turkeys and geese to produce meat or eggs for food originating in the agricultural period. According to the World Watch Institute, 74% of meat consumed worldwide is from poultry meat, and 68% of eggs are derived intensively from poultry, while more than 60 billion chickens are killed annually for consumption [2]. There is little doubt that the demand and therefore the production of poultry will continue to increase relative to the world population, the economy and also the increase in the production of poultry wastes. Poultry waste is used as manure in many fields, but when disposed of in a water body without treatment, it may cause significant problems for aquatic life due to the presence of heavy metals in it. Poultry waste as a mixture of different media involving feces, bedding materials, wasted feeds and feathers, represent favorable media for wide range of chemical and biological hazards include many food-borne pathogens like *Salmonella, Campylobacter, Listeria, Actinomycets, Escherichia coli* and *Clostridium* at high concentrations could reach up to $10^{\hat{}10}$ CFU/gram [3].

3. Trace/heavy metals used as a supplement in poultry feed

Due to increased demand for livestock meats and eggs, there is also a need for increased use of trace elements (some of which are also heavy metals') as nutritional supplements in poultry diets to boost feed quality, promote weight gain and prevent disease, resulting in increased concentration of trace elements added to poultry diets. However, poultry feeds, whether natural or locally sourced or improved by special manufacturing processes, have been reported to be affected by the content of heavy metals in the feed [4]. Many heavy metals are also added to poultry feed as supplements, including copper (Cu), manganese (Mn), iron (Fe), selenium (Se), zinc (Zn) which are important nutrients needed for various biochemical and physiological functions in species, and a lack of supply of these micronutrients results in a number of deficiency diseases or syndromes [5]. Iron and Cu are added to prevent anemia, selenium is added to prevent oxidative cell damage, and Zn and Mn are added to ensure proper egg shell deposition and feather growth [5]. Calcium ($Ca^{2+)}$ is added for bone formation, while in mature laying fowl the majority of dietary calcium is used for egg formation and plays a role in blood clotting and intracellular communication. Antioxidants are added to delay the deterioration of vitamins in poultry feed and tranquilizers may be used to keep flocks quiet in the house and during transport to another pen. A wide variety of antimicrobial drugs are commonly administered to poultry feed as prophylaxis and/or growth promoter and most of the oral applied antibiotics are poorly absorbed in the poultry gut, and then consequently those large amounts of antibiotics were excreted in feces and urine to the environment. Approximately 90% of the applied antibiotics might be excreted as the parent compound [6]. The most common antibiotics such as bactracin, chlortetracycline, monesin, tylosin, penicillin, chloramphenicol and virginiamycin can be applied to poultry feed to fight diseases, pests and increase the

Trace/heavy metals	FAO/WHO [7] and EU [9–12]	National Research council [8]	
	Metals requirement in total diet dry (mg/kg)	Metals requirement in normal diet (ppm)	Toxic level in total diet (ppm)
Cadmium	1 mg/kg		
Chromium	0.01 mg/kg		
Cobalt	1 mg/kg		
Copper	100 mg/kg	6–8 ppm	250–800 ppm
Iron	45–80 mg/kg	50–80 ppm	4,500 ppm
Iodine		0.3–0.4 ppm	625 ppm
Lead	1–5 mg/kg		
Manganese	20–60 mg/kg		
Molybdenum		3–5 ppm	20–10 ppm
Mercury	0.5 mg/kg		
Nickel	0.05 mg/kg		
Selenium		5–20 pm	
Zinc	600 mg/kg	40–75 ppm	800–4,000 ppm

Table 1.
Permissible limits of trace/heavy metals requirements as an additive in poultry feed.

Trace mineral	Egg Layer				Brolier			Brolier Breeder				Cockerel	
	Chick Mash (0–8 Weeks)	Grower Mash (9–17 Weeks)	Layer 1 (18–45 Weeks)	Layer 2 (46–72 Weeks)	Pre-Starter (0–8 Days)	Starter (9–21 Days)	Finisher (22–42 Days)	Broiler Breeder Starter (0–8 Weeks)	Broiler Breeder Grower (9–17 Weeks)	Broiler Breeder Female 1 (18–45 Weeks)	Broiler Breeder Female 2 (46–72 Weeks)	Cockerel Starter (0–8 Weeks)	Cockerel Finisher (9 Weeks – Market)
Manganese (mg)	60	60	60	60	60	30	30	60	60	90	90	60	60
Iron (mg)	30	30	30	30	80	60	60	30	30	30	30	30	30
Copper (mg)	6	6	6	6	5	4	4	6	6	12	12	6	6
Zinc (mg)	60	60	60	60	40	35	35	60	60	100	100	60	60
Iodine (mg)	0.5	0.5	0.5	0.5	0.4	0.4	0.4	0.5	0.5	0.5	0.5	0.5	0.5
Selenium (mg)	0.3	0.3	0.3	0.3	0.2	0.1	0.1	0.3	0.3	0.3	0.3	0.3	0.3

Source: SON [8].

Table 2.
Trace mineral requirements for chicken (per kg of finished feed) mineral.

supply of certain nutrients that transferred through the food chain to humans that induce antimicrobial resistance in humans. Topical pesticides are used as a repellent against flies, lice, bugs, mice and reptiles that can harm or destroy them. WHO/FAO [7], NRC [8], EU [9–12] and SON [13] set acceptable levels of metals in animals, but excessive or deficient use of these metals may lead to deformity in the body or to health problems, some of which may cause serious toxicity, which may lead to the death of the animal (**Tables 1** and **2**). However, pollutants from poultry waste can have detrimental environmental consequences (air, soil and water) if their waste is poorly handled or untreated prior to disposal in the aquatic setting. The disposal of waste produced by the poultry industry is a long-standing concern due to the contribution of nutrients or as a source of heavy metal contamination to our water bodies. Livestock manure may be used as fertilizer in the agricultural sector, it may also degrade the quality of the environment, especially surface and ground water, if it is not properly managed [14]. Untreated poultry waste can degrade water quality when discharged directly to surface water by runoff. The key environmental and health threats associated with animal waste are the introduction of toxins into water sources, such as nutrient limitation (nitrogen and phosphorus), organic matter, sediments, bacteria and heavy metals, which have harmful effects on the living organism and change the nature of the water. However, all mineral elements, whether considered to be necessary or potentially harmful, can have an adverse food impact on humans and animals if they are included in the diet at an overly high concentration [15]. Trace mineral bioavailability is characterized as the proportion of the component consumed that is used for biochemical or physiological purposes [16]. In order to have a high bioavailability, the mineral component must be readily absorbed and rapidly integrate by the body. Bioavailability is mainly influenced by the chemical form of the mineral or the amount in the diet, the amount in the body of the animal, the concentration of other minerals in the diet, its age and the physiological state of the animal to which it is fed. The risk lies in the accumulation of manure-borne metals, as they are not biodegradable and ultimately become phytotoxic, and the long-term use of poultry waste on the soil could lead to the accumulation of heavy/trace elements that increase the potential bioavailability and toxicity of metals in the environment. Such accumulation has the potential to limit soil function, contaminate water and cause toxicity to plants, animals and humans via the food chain. Their bioavailability is determined by physical, chemical and biological factors such as temperature, adsorption, sequestration, lipid solubility and water partition coefficients, whereas biological factors such as species characteristics, trophic interactions and biochemical/physiological adaptation also play an important role [17]. Poultry waste is more toxic than other animal waste due to the high concentration of heavy metals in poultry feed which is not directly absorbed by the body of the animal and egestion as a waste product, while the land application of poultry manure may result in the absorptions of toxicants by plants, animals and humans through absorption, ingestion, bioaccumulation or other processes.

4. Heavy/or trace metals

The word heavy/or trace metals is sometimes used loosely, as they contain a number of metals, some of which are not heavy and some of which are not metals. Heavy metals are a wide class of inorganic chemicals that are harmful to both human and environmental health. Heavy metals are commonly referred to as metals with a minimum density of more than 5 gm/cm3 and adversely impacting the environment and living organisms. Heavy metals include all metals and metalloids except alkali and alkaline earth elements. Some heavy metals are necessary for enzymatic activity and can inhibit enzyme activity when natural concentrations are exceeded. Although some heavy metals are needed as micronutrients, they may be toxic at higher levels than their requirements. In addition, elements such as C, H, O, N, P, S, K, Ca and Mg are often required by majority of species in very small amounts. These elements are called trace elements, such as Fe, Mn, Cu, Co and Mo, and are usually considered to be necessary for most organisms, although V, B and Zn are confirmed to be essential in at least some cases. Most of these trace elements function in an enzyme or in an active group in an enzyme. Since heavy metals cannot be degraded, they are deposited, assimilated or incorporated into water, soil and marine organisms, causing heavy metal contamination in water bodies. Essentials include iron, copper, zinc, cobalt, manganese, chromium, molybdenum, selenium, tin, nickel and vanadium. The deficiency or elevation of these elements can affect the body's normal physiological activities and biochemical processes, resulting in abnormal cell metabolism, development, reproductive disorder and severe oxidative. Non-essential metals are lead, cadmium and mercury. Cobalt, copper, chromium, iron, manganese, nickel, molybdenum, selenium, tin and zinc, sometimes known as trace metals. As a result, the majority of heavy metals, whether necessary or not, are potentially harmful to all living organisms, depends on many factors, such as dosage intake, species chemical composition, age of organisms, gender, genetic make-up and nutritional status of exposed individuals [17]. They have various effects on species depending on dosage exposure and durations of consumption: acute poisoning occurs when exposed to high doses over a short period of time, and chronic poisoning or bioaccumulation occurs when exposed to low doses over a long period of time. 'Toxic metals, including 'heavy metals, 'are individual metals and metal products that have harmful human health effects either by direct or indirect exposure. Trace minerals or heavy metals used in animal feed are often expressed either as parts per million (ppm) or as milligrams per kilogram (mg/kg) of dietary dry matter. In very small quantities, many of these metals are required to sustain life and become toxic in large quantities. They can build ups in biological systems and become a major health hazard" [18]. The term heavy metal refers to any metallic chemical elements that have a comparatively high densities compared to water and are found in traces in different matrices. Their heaviness and toxicity are interrelated as heavy metals are capable of causing toxic or toxic at low concentrations and, if present in animal feed, pose significant health hazards to poultry meat consumers due to biomagnification effects in the body of the animal [19–22]. Heavy metals are normal components of the earth's crust that are not depleted or damaged in the atmosphere and are harmful to human health because they appear to be bioaccumulate for a long period of time, e.g. mercury (Hg), cadmium (Cd), arsenic (As), chromium (Cr), thallium (Tl) and lead (Pb). Bioaccumulation refers to the rise in the concentration of the chemical in the body of the organism over time as opposed to the chemical concentration in the atmospheres. Accumulation of compounds in the organism at any time taken up is processed faster than broken down (metabolized) or excreted. Toxicity could result from any heavy metal, but ten (10) of them are among the top twenty hazardous substances considered to be toxic by several agencies due to their health implications, including arsenic, cadmium, chromium, cobalt, copper, iron, lead, manganese, mercury and platinum [17, 23]. In recent decades, the levels of these metals have risen in our environments as a result of human inputs and activities [24–26]. There are 35 different metals that are of considerable concern to human health due to residential or industrial exposure. They are widely present in the environment and animal diet as a food supplement and are needed in small quantities to maintain good health, but in larger amounts they become harmful or unsafe due to their accumulation in the animal's body over time and may cause serious illness or death. Considering the great variety of heavy metals in the environment, their concentration in various feed chains, it is difficult to achieve a lower level of toxicity than the detection limit for all elements in all products [27]. The European Union, the United States, Asia and other countries are aware of all these problems and as a result numerous laws have been implemented to regulate all heavy metal contamination, reduce the risk of human exposure in the food chain and develop detection methods to control these pollutants in the food chain [28].

The most popular toxic heavy metals are the following: Arsenic (As), Lead (Pb), Mercury (Hg), Cadmium (Cd), Nickel (Ni) and Iron (Fe).

4.1 Arsenic (As)

Arsenic is used in poultry production for growth promotion and for controlling intestinal parasites in which they are fed with arsenic compound called roxarsone (3-nitro-4-hydroxyphenylarsonic acid) while three-quarters of arsenic in feed will be excreted out as poultry waste into environment [29]. Arsenic is a natural soil constituents with concentrations of up to 500 mg/kg. In its essential form, arsenic is insoluble in water, but many of the arsenates are highly soluble. Much if not all-natural water contains compounds of arsenic. Arsenic is the most common cause of acute heavy metal poisoning in adults and is number 1 in the Top 20 List of ATSDR. Arsenic can also be present in water sources worldwide, contributing to contamination of shellfish, cod and haddock. The target organs are the blood, kidney, central nervous, digestive and skin systems [30]. Arsenic is noted for its human toxicity when ingestion of as little as 100 mg typically results in serious poisoning and 130 mg has been shown to be fatal [31]. Several incidents have shown that arsenic in water can be carcinogenic, that skin and probably liver cancers are due to arsenic in drinking water [32, 33].

4.2 Lead (Pb)

Lead is number 2 on the "Top 20 List." for the ATSDR. Lead accounts for most cases of pediatric heavy metal poisoning [30]. Goal organs are bone, brain, blood, kidney, and thyroid gland [23, 34]. Some natural water contains as much as 0.8 mg/l of lead in solution [35]. These concentrations are also found in mountain streams that flow through limestone and galena. It causes acute and chronic toxicity and causes a wide variety of physiological, biochemical and behavioral dysfunctions in humans, animals and aquatic species. Addition of lead to the diet results in a dose-related rise in the concentration of Pb in different organs in the body of animals such as the kidney, blood stream, liver and tibia. It induces oxidative stress that suppresses growth efficiency and decreases feed intake and body weight loss.

4.3 Mercury (Hg)

The number 3 of ATSDR's "Top 20 List" is mercury and naturally generated in the environment by degassing the earth's crust, by volcanic emissions [36]. It is available in three forms: elemental mercury, organic and inorganic mercury. Atmospheric mercury is spread across the globe by winds and returns to the planet in runoff, collecting in marine food chains and fish in lakes [37]. Many researchers believe that dental amalgam could be due to a source of mercury toxicity. Mercurochrome and merthiolate are still in use in drugs, while algaecides are the main possible sources of mercury by inhalation. The organic form is readily absorbed in the gastrointestinal tract (90–100%); Less but nevertheless large amounts of inorganic mercury are absorbed in gastrointestinal tract (7–15%) and the target organs are majorly brain and kidneys [30].

4.4 Cadium (Cd)

Cadmium is a derivative from the smelting or mining activities of lead and zinc in environment and it occupied 7 position on ATSDR's "Top 20 list." It also used in nickel cadmium batteries production, PVC plastics, and paint pigments industries. It can also find in Cigarettes, as well as in soil as a result of insecticides, fungicides, sludge, and other commercial fertilizers that contain cadmium compound in agriculture or in reservoirs that contain shellfish. Other sources of cadmium contamination are from dental alloys, electroplating, engine oil and automobile exhaust. Inhalation of cadmium accounts for 15–50 per cent of assimilate into the respiratory tracts; 2–7 per cent of the ingested cadmium is absorbed into the gastrointestinal system while main target organs are the liver, placenta, kidneys, lungs, brain and bones [30]. Cadmium is moderately harmful to all species and is a cumulative toxin in mammals. In low concentrations, the use of trivalent chromium as an additive in animal diets may induce rapid growth for the animal in order to improve the quality of the meat produced, but often poultry owners may add trivalent chromium in excesses for rapid growth of their animals in order to obtain further value, which may have adverse effects on animals such as those injured and poisonous to the animal. It appears to be concentrated in the kidneys, liver, pancreas and thyroid of humans and other mammals. Humans can be exposed to this metal mainly through inhalation and ingestion, and can suffer from acute and chronic intoxication. Kar and Patra [38] reported that the Cd concentration sometimes increases in feeds, fodders, water bodies, and tissues of livestock which causes metabolic, structural, and functional changes of different organs of all animals. In poultry birds, bioaccumulation of Cd occurs in several organs mainly in the liver, kidney, lung, and reproductive organs due to its continuous exposure. Intake of Cd reduces growth and egg laying performance and feed conversion efficiency in poultry. Chronic exposure of Cd at low doses can also alter the microscopic structures of tissues, particularly in the liver, kidney, brain, pancreas, intestine, and reproductive organs due to increased contents of Cd in these tissues. Continuous Cd exposure causes increased oxidative stresses at cellular levels due to over-production of reactive oxygen species, exhausting antioxidant defense mechanisms. This leads to disruption of biologically relevant molecules, particularly nucleic acid, protein and lipid, and subsequently apoptosis, cell damage, and necrotic cell death. The histopatholocal changes in the liver, kidneys, and other organs are adversely reflected in hemogram and serum biochemical and enzyme activities.

4.5 Iron (Fe)

Iron does not appear on the ATSDR's "Top 20 List, " but it is a heavy metal of concerns, particularly because ingesting dietary iron supplements may acutely poison young children. Uses of Fe as additives in feed formation have many disadvantages such as low bioavailability, high hydroscopicity and oxidative, high excretion and so on [39]. Iron deficiency is still a major problem in several segments of the livestock production causes microcytic, hypochromic anemia in chickens. Iron also plays a role in other enzymes involved in oxygen transport and the oxidative process, including catalase, peroxidases, flavoprotein enzymes and cytochromes. Approximately two-thirds of body iron is found in hemoglobin (red blood cells and myoglobin in the muscles), while 20% is present in labile forms in the liver, spleen and other tissues, with the remainder not available in tissues such as myosin and actmysin and in metalloenzymes. The iron in hemoglobin is essential for the proper function of every organ and tissue of the body. The iron requirement of chicks fed casein, dextrose, and isolated soybean protein concentrate-based diet was studied by Aoyagi and Baker [40]. Ingestion accounts for most of the toxic effects of iron because iron is absorbed rapidly in the gastrointestinal tract and other target organs are the liver, cardiovascular system, and kidneys [30].

4.6 Zinc (Zn)

Zinc plays an important role in biological process in animal including immune function, growth, development and reproduction. It is component of many enzymes contributing in the energy metabolism, protein synthesis and degradation biosynthesis of nuclei acids, carbon dioxide, transport and many more. Its performance major role as an antioxidant in diet, growth and development, production, immunity and stress related issues. It is important in animal diets formation because it influences economic profitability of egg modifying. Zinc has a beneficial impacts on the growth and reproduction of livestock. Due to the low zinc and copper contents of some home-grown feeds compared to guidelines and varying bioavailability, supplementation of these metals is essential for most livestock species and is usually added as mineral supplements to dairy rations [7, 9, 10]. Zinc deficiency causes growth retardation and irregular production of feathers in poultry animals. Feather spattering occurs towards the end of the feather while severity of the spattering ranges from no feathers on the wings and tail to minor defects in the growth of some of the barbels and the hog joint may be widened. Zinc deficiency can causes the long bones of the legs and wings to be shortened and thickened. Other signs include loss of appetite, decreased feed use quality, and death in extreme cases. Zinc deficiencies in the breeding diet decreases egg production and hatchability. Embryos developed in zinc-deficient eggs display a wide range of skeletal anomalies in the head, limbs and vertebrae. The hatched chicks will also not stand, eat or drink [41]. Proper zinc supplementation has been shown to be effective in reducing the early mortality of poultry animals and zinc supplementation is typically applied to animal diets in the form of zinc oxide or zinc sulfate. Latest comparisons of bioavailability in chicks suggest that feed grade zinc oxide has just 44–78 per cent of zinc sulfate availability when added to refined or functional diets [42–44]. Zinc toxicities can cause health problems, and prolonged consumption can also lead to negative side effects such as nausea and vomiting, loss of appetite, diarrhea, abdominal cramping and immunity. The risk associated with zinc deficiency could cause gastrointestinal diseases such as Crohn's disease, decreased immunity, thinning of hair, decreased appetite, weight loss, skeletal malformations, poor bone mineralization, immunological dysfunction, mood disorders, dry skin, fertility problems and impaired wound healing, inadequate dietary intake, poor absorption, genetic mutations. Symptoms of extreme zinc deficiency include impaired growth and development, delayed sexual maturity, chronic diarrhea, impaired wound healing and behavioral problems [45, 46].

4.7 Nickel (Ni)

Nickel is an essential element required in low amount for animal growth and it is required for activities of vitamin B12 and biotin during metabolism of odd-chain fatty acids in animals [47]. Depending on the dose and length of exposure, as an immunotoxic and carcinogen agent, nickel can cause several health problems such as contact dermatitis, cardiovascular disease, asthma, lung fibrosis, and respiratory tract cancer [48, 49]. However, the exposure of human beings mainly concerns oral ingestion through water and food as nickel may be a contaminant in drinking water and/or food [50]. Although the molecular mechanisms of nickel-induced neurotoxicity are not yet clear, oxidative stress and mitochondrial dysfunction have a significant role to play. Mitochondrial nickel-induced damage can occur due to impaired mitochondrial membrane potential, decreased mitochondrial ATP concentration and degradation of mitochondrial DNA [51]. Nickel, high concentrations of which can affect human health badly, can accumulate on plants, animals, and soil.

5. Other trace/heavy metals use as a supplement to prevent deficiency in poultry animals

Copper is necessary for the action of enzymes associated with the metabolism of iron, elastin and collagen formation, melanin production, and the integrity of the central nervous system [41]. Normal red blood cell formation is needed by enabling the absorption of iron from the small intestine and the release of iron into the blood plasmas in the tissue [41]. Copper is necessary for bone formation by promoting the structural integrity of bone collagen and the normal formation of elastin in the cardiovascular system. It needed normal myelination of brain cells and spinal cord as a component of the enzyme cytochrome oxidase, which is necessary for the formation of myelin. Maximum immune response also depends on copper, as shown by depressed titers in deficient animals [41]. The minimum requirement for copper cannot be provided with great precision, because the absorption and utilization of coppers in animals can be significantly influenced by many mineral elements and other dietary factors. The process of natural hair and wool pigmentation includes the use of copper. Copper is believed to be a portion of polyphenyl oxidase that catalyzes the conversion of tyrosine to melanin and the incorporation of disulfide groups into keratin in wool and hair. Copper deficiency causes microcytic, hypochromic anemia, bone weakness, deformity and depigmentation in animals. In copper deficient chicks, aneurysm dissects the aorta, and in other species, cardiac hypertrophy occurs. Copper deficiency in laying hen causes anemia and the development of eggs that are abnormal in size and shape, and some eggs have wrinkled and rough shells [12].

Molybdenum is an essential nutrient because it is a constituent of the enzyme xanthine oxidase and other enzymes. When there is excess molybdenum in animal feeds it causes a copper deficiency which can results in extreme diarrhea, weight loss, bone and joint disorders, affect reproduction and heart function and anemia. Molybdenum has been shown to be essential for growth of animals such as lambs, chicks, and turkey fed highly purified diets. At this time, however, the Food and Drug Administration does not recognize molybdenum use as safe, and current regulations prohibit adding it to animal feed [52, 53].

Manganese was first recognized as a part of necessary nutrient required for growth of animals in the early 1930s, because it is found in many different animal feeds, the effect of its deficiency is less likely than with most of the other trace minerals. The highest manganese concentration can store in the body of animals such as in bone, kidney, liver, pancreas, and pituitary gland. Manganese deficiency in the diet of growing animas like chicks causes perosis, or slipped tendon but it deficient in chicks have less proteoglycan in the cartilage of the tibial growth which twisting and bending of the tibia, and slipping of the gastrocnemius tendon from its condyles [44]. With increase in severity, the chicks are reluctant to move, squat on their stools, and can lead to death of the animal. Lack of manganese breeding or in laying birds can lead to reduce in egg production, hatchability and reduced egg shell strength. In certain cases, most embryos that die due to manganese deficiency display chondrodystrophy which is a disorder characterized by a parrot-like beak, wire and shortening of long bones [41].

Iodine combined with tyrosine in the thyroid to form diiodotyrosine. Iodine deficiency in breeding hens could result in reduced egg iodine levels, reduced egg development, decreased hatchability, extended hatching period, and increased embryos in the thyroid gland. Goiter develops in the thyroid gland, which causes the thyroids gland to expand to several times its usual size. Histological analysis of the thyroid has indicated hyperplasia and lack of colloid. The thyroid gland contains the highest concentration (0.2 per cent to 5 per cent on a dry weight basis) of iodine in the body; 70 per cent to 80 per cent of the total body stocks. Approximately 90 percent of the iodine that passes through the thyroid gland is captured by that organ [54]. Two molecules of this compound are then mixed to form tyroxine. Approximately 80 per cent of the thyroxine entering the circulation is broken down by de-iodization of the liver, kidneys and other tissues.

Selenium is one of the most commonly known nutrient deficiencies in animal growth and was recognized as a potentially harmful mineral until it was identified as an essential nutrient. It plays a significant role in the preventing exudative diatheses in chicks and is present in all cells of the body while the concentration is generally less than 1 ppm but its harmful absorption in liver and kidneys are usually ranged between 5 and 10 ppm. Selenium is a crucial component of enzyme glutathione peroxidase that eliminate peroxide compounds from the body tissues and it essential in the synthesis of sulfur amino acids that helps in protecting animals from a variety of diseases associated with low intakes of selenium and vitamin E. Selenium and vitamin E are both effective antioxidants that prevent peroxide from destroying the body cells. Selenium can be added to the diet of all food animals. Birds may be fed up to 0.1 ppm of selenium in the total diet, whereas excess selenium in animal diets must be avoided if sufficient precautions are taken in addition to animal diets. All these animals need selenium at a level of 0.1 ppm in the total diets (except the turkey, which requires 0.2 ppm, and the baby pig, 0.3 ppm). Generally higher levels of protein, sulfur and arsenic can partly protect against the toxicity of excess selenium. Selenium is quickly extracted from the body of the infected animals when the animal is fed selenium-low [55]. In broilers feed with diet containing low selenium e.g., chickens of 3 to 6 weeks begin to display signs of weight loss, weakening of the leg and eventual lead to death. Extreme deficiency of selenium is shown with the sign of growth retardation and the mortality rate rise even in the presence of sufficient vitamin E. Disease like Pancreatic fibrosis, reduction of pancreatic output of lipase, chymotrypsinogen and trypsinogen are related to selenium deficiency. Pancreatic lesions disease arises as early as 6 days old chicken and typically return to normal within two weeks when selenium is used as a feed supplementation in their diet. The most sensitive requirements for selenium deficiency are egg hatchability in laying hens. Selenium results from encephalomalacia, membrane lipid peroxidation, erythrocyte hemolysis and muscular dystrophies [41].

6. Recent research on the quality of heavy metals in poultry feed

Based on the study by Eloma et al. [56], which analyzed six potentially toxic elements (PTEs) from poultry feeds such as Cd, Cr, Cu, Pb, Mn, Ni and Zn, four feed forms (starter, grower, finisher and layer) from four producers coded A, B, C and D were sold in Ebony State, Nigeria. The mean concentrations of metals recorded from poultry feeds were as following: Chromium (11.9–7.90 mg/kg); Copper (5.10–7.91 mg/kg); Cadmium (0.49–0.76 mg/kg); Lead (7.17–9.47 mg/kg); Manganese (26.9–34.9 mg/kg); Nickel (3.80–6.50 mg/kg) and Zinc (27.8–38.4 mg/kg). The result of these findings was compared with European Union standard of PTEs maximum acceptable concentration in feed while Pb and Ni concentrations were above the maximum acceptable limits that is risk to human health. Thus, there is a need for continuous monitoring of feed compositions. Lead and Ni exceeded permissible limits by European Union in feed as stipulated, but the perilous elements such as Cr, Cu and Zn were also high in feed. There is however a need for continuous monitoring of feed compositions and also for the introduction of practices that will not introduce PTEs into the system. It also recommended that a proximate study be carried-out on poultry feeds to determine its moisture content, ash content, crude fiber, lipid, crude protein, carbohydrate and metabolizable energy [57–59].

Kabir and Bhuyan [60] were conducted to determine the heavy metal content of hens (*Gallus gallus domesticus*) and ducks (*Anas platyrhynchos*) from the Chittagong regions of Bangladesh. Chromium (Cr) and cadmium (Cd) concentrations were found below the detection limit in both hens and ducks of the egg. The concentrations of Iron (Fe) ranged from 58.4 to 78.90 mg/kg was recorded for hen and duck yolks and 3.90 to 11.62 mg/kg for albumin. The highest concentration was recorded in hen layer eggs (78.90 mg/kg), while the lowest concentration was observed in native duck eggs (58.4 mg/kg). The highest concentration of 11.62 mg/kg was recorded from albumin of indigenous duck eggs, while the lowest of 3.90 mg/kg was observed in indigenous hen eggs. The copper concentration ranged from 1.85 to 3.95 mg/kg was recorded from hen and duck yolk, while in albumin these amounts ranged from 0.25 to 1.15 mg/kg. The highest value (3.95 mg/kg) of indigenous hen eggs was reported, while the lowest concentration was 1.85 mg/kg for hen eggs. The highest concentration of 1.15 mg/kg was reported in albumin of domestic duck eggs, while the lowest value of 0.25 mg/kg was observed from native hen eggs. There was significant difference in the concentrations of Fe ($p = 0.00$) and Cu ($p = 0.00$) in both yolk and albumin. However, there were no major variations in the number of Fe ($p = 0.998$) and Cu ($p = 0.458$) in terms of the animal type (indigenous hen, indigenous duck, layer hen).

Korish and Attia [61] conducted research on heavy metal content in feed, litter, meat, meat products, liver and table eggs of chickens. Concentrations of heavy metals were examined in chicken meat, meat products, feed, litter, as well as laying hen eggs to track the regularity of this metals in the market products and their protection for human consumption as recommended daily allowance (RDA). Samples were collected from most popular poultry products in Saudi Arabia. A total of 45 samples from frozen broiler meat, fresh beef, liver, frankfurter and burger were collected from the same brand. However, 60 table eggs were collected from four different commercial brands while the edible parts of egg were analyzed to determine the levels of mineral elements present in it. In addition, 30 samples from different feed and litter were collected from the starter feed, grower feed, diets of layer broilers and laying hens. The findings showed that there were extensive amounts of most trace or heavy metals in the various meat sources while liver had the highest concentration of all elements examined, except for Co, Cr and Ni. The highest amount of Chromium concentration was recorded in fresh meat, followed by frozen meat. Trace or heavy metals such as Mn, Co, Ni and Pb were not detected in frozen or fresh meat. The chicken burger and the frankfurter samples have similar concentrations of trace/heavy metal except for Zn and Mn which had higher concentrations was observed in frankfurter compared to burger sample. There were significant differences between zinc concentration of the different sources of eggs. Fe was significantly higher in beef meat compared to poultry meat but the opposite trend for Zn was observed. All heavy metals concentration in were higher in liver than the eggs, except for Chromium while the burger had higher concentrations of Cu and Co. finally, it concluded that Cd, Pb, As and Se are not detected in chicken meat and eggs produced which indicate that no human hazards from these toxic elements.

However, the liver had the highest concentration of all heavy metals examined, except for Cr, and the intake of Pb and Cd from the broiler liver was higher than the RDA for adults. Burgers and frankfurters, showed higher concentrations of Pb, Cd and Ni than chicken meat and table eggs, implying a potential human health danger. Therefore, in order to enhance the quality of poultry products for human consumption, adequate legislation is required to regulate the quality of poultry products, as well as feed/food and chicken litter. In addition, critical measurements should be used for the detoxification of heavy metals from waste. The relationship between the minerals in poultry production and the diet of poultry and poultry litter remains fertile for further study.

Study of Dahri et al. [62] on the investigation of concentrations of heavy metals; lead and chromium in chicken feed collected from commercial poultry feed markets and local poultry farms in Hyderabad Sindh. A total of eight samples of poultry feeds, four of which were commercial feed samples and four of which were local feed samples collected in polyethylene bags. The samples were analyzed using the Aurora Al1200 Atomic Absorption Spectrophotometer (AAS) for heavy metals; lead (Pb) and chromium (Cr). Relatively higher concentrations of lead (Pb) have been found in commercial feed samples. Data obtained from the present study for lead and chromium beyond the allowable limit, i.e., 0.05 and 0.1 ppm as recommended by WHO/FAO. Lead (Pb) and chromium (Cr) metals are important for the growth of poultry, but they may become toxic if the concentrations exceed the allowable limits. Excessive quantities of metals taken by animals make their way to the human body, which is extremely dangerous to human health. Heavy metal contamination is prevalent in the Hyderabad district and thus in the present report, the amount of poultry feed is alarming. The nutritional values of the feed are therefore calculated from the concentrations of lead and chromium above the allowable level in the feed content.

7. Causes of heavy metal contamination in the body of water

Aquatic ecosystems are highly complex, diverse and subject to a variety of internal and external relationships that are subject to change over time. Public health issues are among the pollutants that the concentration of heavy metals in marine environments enters humans through food chains. Heavy metal contamination may occur from many causes, but most generally results from metal purification, e.g., copper smelting and nuclear fuel preparation. Following the introduction of heavy metal pollutants into the flow, whether from natural or anthropogenic sources, they divide between aqueous (pore water and overlying water) and solid phases (sediment, suspended particulate matter and biota). Anthropogenic metals can persistently persist inside water bodies, or these elements are absorbed by silt, likely absorbed by animals, and accumulate in the food chain, beginning easily with plankton, such as filtering zooplankton, benthos, or fish, and eventually transferred to humans. Unlike organic contaminants that lose biodegradation toxicity, heavy metals cannot be degraded/decayed and thus pose a different form of remediation challenge. Heavy metals such as lead, mercury, iron, cadmium, aluminum and magnesium are found in water supplies. If these metals are found in the sediment, they enter the food chain through plants and aquatic animals. **Impact of heavy metals on aquatic organisms.**

The effects of heavy metals on marine species vary from a small drop in the rate of growth to death. Pollutants entering inshore waters and estuaries cause severe problems, causing significant harm to the life and activities of living aquatic species and also to the mass mortality of organisms. The gradual and irreversible accumulation of these metals in the various organs of the creatures of life contributes to long-term metal-related diseases due to their toxicity, endangering aquatic biota and other organisms [36]. Heavy metal pollution may have detrimental effects on the ecological balance of the recipient ecosystem and the diversity of marine species [63–65]. Among the animal species, fish are those that cannot avoid the adverse effects of these contaminants [66–68]. These metals are responsible not only for the deterioration of the water quality of the body, but also for the death of a variety of aquatic species [69]. The disposal of these wastes adversely affects water bodies, changes their chemical composition and causes harm to both humans and aquatic organisms [70–72]. These heavy metals (arsenic, cadmium, chromium, cobalt, copper, iron, lead, manganese, mercury and platinum) become toxic by accumulations of flora and fauna in the body tissues and then move through the food chain from fish to humans [73, 74]. Cadmium causes certain problems similar to those caused by mercury, which are much more harmful than mercury; Daphina, Scenedesmus and *E. coli* are very susceptible [69]. Some of these heavy metals are important to human metabolism while some are dangerous, particularly when their concentrations are higher [75, 76]. The presences of heavy metals observed in most of marine animals is becoming a threats to human health, rendering them unfit for human consumption [1]. The presences of lethal metals in ecological environments are one of the key concerns of pollution control and environmental interventions in most parts of the world [77, 78]. Copper is more widely recorded as an algal toxin in contaminated waters than as a restricting algal growth [79]. Freshwater animals are probably more susceptible based on the estimates that 50 per cent of the waterfowl population of Daphina magna died at concentrations between 25 and 65 μg/l, the exact values depending on the experimental exposure period and age of the animals. Ionic copper tends to be a real toxic material, whereas oxides or other colloidal particles or chelates are much less dangerous. In general, mollusks and fish tolerate higher concentrations of trace metals than other phylae studied. Acute and sub-lethal effects of zinc pollution on aquatic ecosystems have been extensively studied among different species of fish [80]. The toxicity of zinc to fish has been shown to depend on the nature of the water. Acute toxicity is increased by the rise in water temperature and the resulting reduction in oxygen content.

Mercury emission experiments in aquatic environments indicate that recovery from pollution will take place within a limited period of time following the cessation of pollution input [81]. The embryonic and larval stages of marine organisms are typically the most susceptible periods of the life cycle for heavy metals and other toxicants. Copper accelerated the mortality of *Mytilus edulis* during the reproductive cycle and impaired respiration by destroying the respiratory membranes. Mercury has often been seen with curiosity and alarm. It's the only metal that's liquid at a regular temperature (hence its other name, quicksilver) and it fun to play with. Its vapor is toxic and can vaporize quickly enough to be lethal at high temperatures). Any of its compounds, the toxicity of which has been well known since the Middle Ages, have been used as agents of murder and suicide. However, until quite recently, mercury was not considered a dangerous water pollutant, since it is harmful in vapor form and is not especially hazardous when taken by mouth as a liquid. Arsenic, lead, cadmium and mercury are cumulative cell poisons with a strong propensities to be deposited in the bone, particularly in the case of lead. The signs of moderate chronic poisoning are not well described and therefore difficult to diagnose. Heavy metals become harmful to the body of an organism when they are not metabolized and accumulate in soft tissues and can reach the human body through food chain, water, air, or absorption through the skin when they come into contact with humans [36].

8. Health hazards pose by poultry waste in an environment

The great concern lies in the excessive accumulation of macro-minerals (Ca, Si, Fe), trace elements (Cu, Mn, Zn, Se), heavy metals (Pb, Hg, Cd), medicinal drugs (antibiotics, coccidiostatics, sulfa drugs, etc.), anti-metabolites, insecticides, herbicides, wood preservatives, mycotoxins and hormones, harmful organisms transmittable other non-nutritional excretory via wastes to man. Poultry waste contains considerable amounts of nutrients (nitrogen and phosphorus) and other excreted substances such as hormones, antibiotics, harmful pathogens and heavy metals. Leaching and runoff of these substances has the potential to contamination both the surface water and/or nearby groundwater (Steinfeld et al., in [82]). Thus, increased outputs of phosphorus and nitrate to fresh water which can caused severe water quality problems like accelerate eutrophication in surface waters due to high inputs of organic substances and nutrients through runoffs which can result into accumulation pollution nutrient-sensitive ecosystems resulting in biodiversity losses such as fish kills due to hypoxia/anoxia and high levels of ammonia, harmful toxic algal blooms, decreases in water clarity, widespread anoxia, declines in submerged aquatic vegetation, shifts in pH, and depletion of oxygen. A drop in the level of dissolved oxygen in surface water has deleterious effects on fish populations [83, 84]. Furthermore, eutrophication can spur the growth of toxic microorganisms, such as *Pfiesteria piscicida*, that have been found to cause temporary memory loss, immuno-suppressions, and decreased cognitive function in exposed populations, respiratory problems and eye irritation, as well as gastroenteritis, headaches, and fatigue [6]. Skin irritation and lesions have also been reported among those with direct contact with contaminated surface waters, particularly among fishermen [6]. The leaching of nitrates and pathogens into water can cause significant cognitive loss and nervous system impairment when ingested by humans [6].

Poultry waste contains toxic metals that are bioaccumulate in the body of aquatic organisms and become biomagnification through food chain to next trophic level which can cause health hazard to human such as arsenic which is carcinogen and may also lead to heart disease, diabetes, and a decline in mental functioning. These harmful bacteria and chemicals present in poultry waste threaten the human health and aquatic organisms globally. Also of concern is the issue of air quality affected by dust particles, releases significant emissions of gases (methane, hydrogen sulfides, sulfur dioxide and ammonia) offensive odors and other pollutants such as volatile organic compounds (VOCs), particulate matter (PM), nitrogenous compounds during the decomposition of poultry waste that contributed to climate change which is a global concern and deleterious health effects (both chronic and acute) including respiratory conditions (i.e., bronchitis, asthma in children), heart disease, and lung cancer [85, 86]. Poultry waste as an important source of nutrients for many edible crops, may also contain some biological hazards that can threaten human health [87]. Poultry waste could be a source of human pathogens such as Salmonella, Campylobacter and Listeria that can potentially contaminate both edible crops and environment, which consequently leads to food-borne diseases [88, 89]. Poultry litter contains wide and diverse counts of microorganism including both of gram positive and negative bacteria. Among the bacterial and fungal species that are biological hazard to human health was recorded from poultry litter and waste such as *Actinobacillus, Bordetella, Campylobacter, Clostridium, Corynebacterium, E. coli, Globicatella, Listeria, Mycobacterium, Salmonella, Staphylococcus,* and *Streptococcus* [6]. Accumulation of high concentration of heavy metals initiates numerous fatal signs including hepato-renal dysfunctions and reproductive complications. Cd toxicity effect can persist more than 10–35 years in the body due to long biological half-life. After absorption, it is primarily stored and distributed in various tissues, primarily, in the liver and kidney. It has been proved that Cd has direct toxic effects on the cellular levels which lead to apoptotic and necrotic cell deaths. It is also responsible for malignant growth and it is categorized as a type 1 carcinogen [38]. Exposure of Cd to livestock including poultry not only affects health, but also hampers animal production reducing growth performance and feed utilization efficiency in their body.

9. Diseases caused by heavy metals

Heavy metal contamination is known to cause numerous diseases worldwide, such as minamata disease (organic mercury poisoning), iltai-itai disease (cadmium poisoning), arsenic acid poisoning, and asthma induced air pollution (Matsuo, 2003). The worst examples of accumulation are recorded in Japan, where hundreds of fishermen were killed by consuming fish containing too much mercury (Minamata Disease, [37]) or cadmium (itai-itai disease Kobayashi, 1971). These tragedies resulted from the tragic coincidence of a predominantly fish-eating and fish-eating population, which while having high concentrations of mercuries, did not show any symptoms. A special feature makes the mercury issue more important because under anaerobic conditions after sedimentation, it can be transformed to yet more toxic methylmercury compounds, which like metals, may accumulate in organisms that are possibly adsorbed to –SH groups in enzymes and even in food chains. Conversion to methylmercury is a bacteriological conversion involving methane bacteria. As a part of this reaction, mercury adsorbed to sediments may be mobilized after they are settled (which would also contribute to anaerobic conditions) and accumulate in fish via food chains. Copper is another aspect that creates concern in contaminated water. Approximately 1 g of copper causes acute illness in humans. Some freshwater algae tend to require either cobalt or vitamin B12. Copper is also less harmful than mercury, and incidents like Minamata are not likely to occur, nor do drinking water appear to be poisoning. Copper disposal is so common and widespread, however that amounts of copper in aquatic environments can typically be high enough to cause harm to species. If humans eat food tainted with heavy metals and their concentrations are amplified because they cannot be excreted. If the concentration exceeds a lethal level, it can results in brain injury or death. Lead affects the central and peripheral nervous systems, organs, bones and kidneys. Lead does not have an advantageous biological role and is believed to store in the body. Lead acquaintance can cause antagonistic effects on human health, particularly in young children and pregnant women, as Pb is a neurotoxin that always disrupts normal brain development. It accumulates in the skeleton, induces bone mobilization during pregnancy, lactation exposure to fetuses and breastfed babies. Cellular and molecular lead can increase the incidence of carcinogenic events associated with DNA damage and suppress DNA repair and tumor controls. Lead is a toxic metal that is particularly harmful to children. Health issues caused by low levels of chronic exposure to heavy metals may take years for humans to develop and may be related to heavy metals [36]. Most of the exposure to heavy metal contamination has been clinically shown to be associated with causing free radical harm leading to: heart attacks, strokes, cancer and several circulatory disorders other than cardiovascular diseases that do not cause death, but may affect the quality of life. Any of these include: Impotence, Asthma, Diabetes, Exhaustion, Alzheimer's Disease, Memory Loss. Lead poisoning is a severe, very common form of heavy metal poisoning and the symptoms of lead poisoning in children are close to those of attention deficit hyperactivity disorder (ADHD). Lead poisoning also 07 triggers behavioral and cognitive disabilities, nervousness, headaches, and many other associated symptoms.

Metals may be extracted from aqueous sources such as chemical precipitation, lime coagulation, ion exchange, reverse osmosis and solvent extraction [90]. Other methods include electrodialysis, ultrafiltration and biosorption; [36]. At present, phytoremediation (plants or microorganisms) is being used at an early stage to extract heavy metals from water, sediment and soil by concentrating them in their organic matter.

10. Conclusion

Increased regular releases of anthropogenic activities such as untreated poultry waste containing heavy metals into the aquatic environment globally, particularly in underdeveloped countries, could pose a risk to aquatic species as well as affect the ecological balance that can be transmitted via the food chain to humans and could pose serious human health problems. Regulation of the use of heavy metals as an additive or complete elimination of heavy metals in animal feed should be carried out in order to mitigate the human health risks associated with the use of animal products and the contamination of the atmosphere by manure. Preventive steps should be taken to minimize the level of heavy metal contamination in the marine ecosystems by destroying animals when the concentration is too high or consumed and transmitted to humans.

Author details

Adesakin Taiwo Adekanmi
Department of Biology, Ahmadu Bello University, Zaria, Nigeria

*Address all correspondence to: ataiwonelson@gmail.com

References

[1] Banerjee, S, Maiti, S. K, and Kumar, A. (2015). Metal contamination in water and bioaccumulation of metals in the plankton, molluscs and fishes in Jamshedpur stretch of Subarnarekha River of Chotanagpur plateau, India. Water and Environment Journal, 29: 207-213.

[2] World Watch Institutes (2006). State of the World *2006*, p. 26.

[3] Bolan, N. S., Adriano, D. C. and Mahimairaja, S. (2004). Distribution and bioavailability of trace elements in livestock and poultry manure by-products. Critical Reviews in Environmental Science and Technology, 34: 291-338.

[4] Islam, M. S, Kazi, M. A. I, Hossain, M. M., Ahsan, M. A. and Hossain, A. M. M. M. (2007): Propagation of heavy metals in poultry feed production in Bangladesh. *Bangladesh Journal of Scientific and Industrial Research*, 42(4): 456-474.

[5] Oyewale, A.T., Adesakin, T.A., Oyedeji, O., Aduwo, A.I. and Bakare, M.K. (2018). Impact Assessment of Poultry Discharge on the Physico-Chemical and Microbiological Water Quality of Olosuru Stream in Ikire, Southwestern Nigeria. *Journal of Water Resource and Protection*, Vol. 10, Pp 1061-1082.

[6] Madgy, S. M. (2017). More Nutrients and more hazards when using poultry litter in Plant and/or Animal Nutrition. *Nutrition and Food Science,* Page 1-5

[7] FAO/WHO (2003). JOINT FAO/WHO food standards programme codex committee on food additives and contaminants: FAO, Nutrition meetings Report series NO. 51A and WHO, Food additive series NO 4. Thirty-sixth Session Rotterdam.

[8] NRC (1994). *Nutrient Requirements of Poultry. 9th revised edition*, National Academy of Sciences, Washington, DC. Pp 19-34.

[9] European Commission (2003a): Opinion of the scientific committee on animal nutrition on undesirable substances in feed. European Commission, Health and Consumer Protection Directorate, Brussels, Belgium.

[10] European Commission (2003b). Opinion of the scientific committee on animal nutrition on the use of zinc in feedstuffs. European Commission, Health and Consumer Protection Directorate, Brussels, Belgium. **2003a**.

[11] European Commission (2003c). Opinion of the scientific committee on animal nutrition on the use of copper in feedstuffs. European Commission, Health and Consumer Protection Directorate, Brussels, Belgium. **2003b**.

[12] European Commission (2003d). Opinion of the scientific committee on animal nutrition on undesirable substances in feed. European Commission, Health and Consumer Protection Directorate, Brussels, Belgium. **2003c**.

[13] SON (2018). Standard for poultry feed by Nigeria Industrial Standard, Plot 13/14 victoria Arobieke street NO.52 Lome Street, pg. 1-48.

[14] Kumar, K., Gupta, S. C., Chander, Y. and Singh, A. K. (2005). Antibiotic Use in Agriculture and Its Impact on the Terrestrial Environment. *Advances in Agronomy*. Vol. 87, Pp 1-54.

[15] Okoye, C. O. B., Ibeto, C. N. and Ihedioha, J. N. (2011). Assessment of heavy metals in chicken feeds sold in south eastern, Nigeria. *Pelagia Research*

Library Advances in Applied Science Research. Vol. 2(3), Pp 63-68.

[16] O'Dell, B.L. (1997). Mineral-ion interaction as assessed by bioavailability and ion channel function. In: B.L. O'Dell and R. A. Sunde (eds.) Handbook of nutritionally essential mineral elements. P. 641. Marcel Dekker, Inc., New York.

[17] Tchounwou, P. B., Yedjou, C. G., Patlolla, A. K. and Sutton, D. J. (2012). Heavy metals toxicity and the environment. Experimental Neurology 101, 133-164.

[18] OSHA (2004). Safety and Health Topics: Toxic Metals. U.S. Dept. of Labour, Occupational Safety and Health (OSHA)

[19] Bhargava, A, Carmona, F. F., Bhargava, M. and Srivastava, S. (2012). Approaches for enhanced phytoextraction of heavy metals. The Journal of Environmental Management, 105, 103-120.

[20] Dai, S. Y., Jones, B, Lee, K. M, Li, W, Post, L. and Herrman, T. J. (2016). Heavy metal contamination of animal feed in Texas. Journal of Regulatory Science 01, 21-32.

[21] Giromini, C, Rebucci, R, Fusi, E, Rossi, L, Saccone, F. and Baldi, A. (2016). Cytotoxicity, apoptosis, DNA damage and methylation in mammary and kidney epithelial cell lines exposed to ochratoxin. Cell Biology and Toxicology, 32, 249-258.

[22] Govind, P. and Madhuri, S. (2014). Heavy metals causing toxicity in animals and fishers. *Research Journal of Animal,* Veterinary and Fishery Sciences Vol. 2, 17-23.

[23] Agency for Toxic Substances and Disease Registry (1992). A public health assessment guidance manual. US Dept. of Health and Human Services, Atlanta, Georgia.

[24] Jaishankar, M, Mathew, B. B, Shah, M. S, Murthy, K and Gowda, K. R. S. (2014a). Biosorption of few heavy metal ions using agricultural wastes. Journal of Environmental Pollution and Human Health 2: 1-6.

[25] Jaishankar, M, Tseten, T, Anbalagan, N, Mathew, B. B. and Beeregowda, K. N. (2014b). Toxicity, mechanism and health effects of some heavy metals. Interdisciplinary Toxicology. 7, 60-72.

[26] Nagajyoti, P. C, Lee, K. D, Sreekanth, T. V. M. (2010). Heavy metals, occurrence and toxicity for plants: a Review. Environmental Chemistry Letters 8: 199-216.

[27] Aragay, G, Pons, J. and Merkoçi, A. (2011). Recent trends in macro-, micro-, and nanomaterial-based tools and strategies for heavy-metal detection. Chemical Reviews 111, 3433-3458.

[28] Erdogan, Z., Erdogan, S. Celik, S., and Unlu, A. (2005). Effects of ascorbic acids on cadmium-induced oxidative stress and performance of broiler. Biological trace element research 104 (1): 19-31.

[29] Kathe, J. (1973). 'Das Arse Vordommen Bei Reichenstein und die sogenannte Reichensteiner Krankheit Jahresbericht der schlesischen Gesellschaft fuer Vaterlaendische Kultr Medizinisch-naturwisenshaft-Lidie Reihe, No, 3 Breslau Ferdinand Wirt.

[30] Roberts, J. R. (1999). Metal toxicity in children. In Training Manual on Pediatric Environmental Health. Emeryville CA: Children's Environmental Health.

[31] Browning, E. (1961). 'Toxicity of industrial metals' Butterworths London, England.

[32] Arguello, R. A., Tello, E. E., Macola, B. A. and Manzan, L. (1960). "Cutaneous cancer in chronic endemic

regional Arsenicism in the province of cordoba Argentine Reublic Rev. Fac. Giec. Med. Univ. Cordoba 8409 (1950); Proc. Conf. on physiological Aspects of water quality, public Health Service.

[33] Tello, E. E. (1951). Hidraarsencism cronico regional endemic Hacre Imrinta de la universidact cordoba Re. Argentina p 162.

[34] International Occupational Safety and Health Information Centre, Metals (1999). In Basics of Chemical Safety. Chapter 7 Geneva. International Labour Organization

[35] Lambou, V. and Lim, B. (1970). Hazards of lead in the environment with particular reference to aquatic environment EWQA US Dept. of interior August 1970 (mimeo).

[36] Joseph, B., Raj, S., Edwin, T. B., Sankarganesh, P., Jeevitha, M. V., Ajisha, S.U. and Sheeja, S. (2010). Toxic effect of heavy metals on aquatic environment. *International Journal of Biological and Chemical Sciences*. Vol. 4(4), Pp 939-952.

[37] Clarkson, T.W. and Magos, L. (2006). The toxicology of mercury and its chemical compounds. Crit. Rev. Toxicol. 36:609-662.

[38] Kar, I. and Patra, A. (2021). Tissue Bioaccumulation and Toxicopathological Effects of Cadmium and its Dietary Amelioration in Poultry-a Review. *Biological Trace Element Research*, page 1-25

[39] Ma, X., Liu, S., Lu, L., Li, S., Xie, J., Zhang, L., Zhang, J. and Luo, X. (2014). Relative bioavailability of Iron proteinate for broilers fed a casein-dextrose diet. Poultry science, 93 (3), 556-563.

[40] Aoyagi, S. and Baker, D.H. (1995): Iron requirement of chicks fed a semi purified diet based on casein and soy protein concentrate. Poultry Science, 74:412.

[41] Berger, L. L. (2006). Salt and Trace minerals for livestock poultry and other animals, Salt Institutes 700 North Fairfax street, suite 600 Alexandria, Virginia 22314-22040.

[42] Larson, C.K., (2005). Role of trace minerals in animal production. Presented at the 2005 Nutrition Conference, Department of Animal Science, University of Tennessee. http://www.tennesseenutritionconference.org/Conference2005.htm.

[43] Sandoval, M., Henry, P.R., Ammerman, C.B., Miles, R.D. and Littell, R.C. (1997). Relative bioavailability of supplemental inorganic zinc sources for chicks. Journal of Animal Science, 75:3195.

[44] Wedekind, K.J., Hortin, A.E. and Baker, D.H. (1992). Methodology for assessing zinc bioavailability: efficacy of estimates for zinc-methionine, zinc sulphate and zinc oxide. Journal of Animal Science, 70:178.

[45] Linnik, P. and Zubenko, I. B. (2000). Role of bottom sediments in the secondary pollution of aquatic environments by heavy-metal compounds. *Lakes Reserved*. Vol. 5(1), Pp 11-21.

[46] Nielsen, J. B., and Grandjean, P. (2000). Mercury. In Morton Lippmann (ed.) Environmental Toxicants: Human Exposures and Their Health Effects, John Wiley and Sons, Inc. pp. 563-575.

[47] Nielsen, F. H. (1991). Nutritional requirement for boron, silicon, vanadium, nickel, and arsenic: Current knowledge and speculation. The FASEB Journal, 5 (12): 2261-2667.

[48] Genchi, G., Carocci, A., Lauria, G., Sinicropi, M. S. and Catalano, A.

(2020). Review: Nickel: Human Health and Environmental Toxicology, Int. J. Environ. Res. Public Health 2020, 17, 679.

[49] Song, X., Kenston, S.S.F., Kong, L. and Zhao, J. (2017). Molecular mechanisms of nickel induced neurotoxicity and chemoprevention. Toxicology, 392, 47-54.

[50] Sinicropi, M.S.; Rovito, N.; Carocci, A.; Genchi, G. (2012). Acetyl-L-carnitine in Parkinson's disease. In Mechanisms in Parkinson's Disease—Models and Treatments; Dushanova, J., Ed.; InTech: London, UK, Chapter 19; pp. 367-392. ISBN 978-953-307-876-2.

[51] Carocci, A., Sinicropi, M.S., Catalano, A., Lauria, G. and Genchi, G. (2014). Melatonin in Parkinson's disease. In ASynopsis of Parkinson's Disease; InTech: London, UK, 2014; Chapter 3; pp. 71-99. ISBN 978-953-51-1229-7.

[52] Prudencio, M. I., Gonzalez, M. I., Dias, M. I., Galan, E. and Ruiz, F. (2007). Geochemistry of sediments from El Melah lagoon (NE Tunisia): a contribution for the evaluation of anthropogenic inputs. *Journal Arid Environment*. Vol. 69(2), Pp 285-298.

[53] Raloff, J. (2003). Food for thought. *Global Food Trends Science.*

[54] Hetzel, B.S. and Welby, M.C. (1997). Iodine. In: O'Dell, B.L. and Sunde, R.A. (eds.) Handbook of Nutritionally Essential Mineral Elements. Marcel Dekker, New York, p 557.

[55] NRC (1985). Nutrient Requirements of Poultry. 8th revised ed. National Academy Press. Washington, D.C.

[56] Eloma, N. I, Nwanji, O. L., Ikelle, I. I., Nworu, J. S. and Chukwu, C. O. (2020). Determination of Potentially Toxic Elements from Poultry Feeds in Ebonyi State, Nigeria. *Acta Chemica Malaysia* (ACMY), 2021, Volume 5, Issue 1.

[57] Mahesar, S. A., Sherazi, S. T. H., Abdul, N. M. I. and Bhanger, S. A. (2010). Simultaneous assessment of zinc, cadmium, lead and copper in poultry feeds by differential pulse anodic striping voltammetry. Food and Chemical Toxicology.

[58] Yousuf, M. H. and El-Shahawi A. (1999). Trace metals in Lethrinus lentjan fish from Arabian Gulf: Metal accumulation in Kidney and Heart Tissues. Bulletin of Environmental Contamination and Toxicology, 62(3): 293-300.

[59] Zhan, G. H. (1998). Animal manure can raise soil pH. Stillwater. *Oklahoma Cooperative Extension Service* Vol. 2.

[60] Kabir, A. and Bhuyan, M. S. (2019). Heavy Metals in Egg Contents of Hens (Gallus gallus domesticus) and Ducks (Anas platyrhynchos) from Chittagong Region, Bangladesh. *J Pollut Eff Cont*, Vol. 7 Iss. 1 No: 232

[61] Korish, M. A., and Attia, Y. A. (2020). Evaluation of Heavy Metal Content in Feed, Litter, Meat, Meat Products, Liver, and Table Eggs of Chickens, Animals, 10, 727 pg 4-22.

[62] Dahri, S., Pathan, A. A., Balouch, A. and Mallah, S. (2019). Assessment of Heavy Metals in Poultry Feed of Hyderabad, Sindh, 2nd International Conference on Sustainable Development in Civil Engineering, MUET, Pakistan (December 05-07, 2019.)

[63] Ashraj W. (2005): Accumulation of heavy metals in kidney and heart tissues of Epinephelus microdon fish from the Arabian Gulf. Environmental Monitoring Assessment, 101(1-3): 311-316.

[64] Farombi, E. O., Adelowo, O. A, and Ajimoko, Y. R. (2007). Biomarkers of oxidative stress and heavy metal levels as indicators of environmental pollution in African Cat fish (*Clarias gariepinus*)

from Ogun River, Nigeria. International Journal of Environment Research and Public Health, 4(2): 158-165.

[65] Vosyliene, M. Z. and Jankaite, A. (2006). Effect of heavy metal model mixture on rainbow trout biological parameters. Ekologija, 4: 12-17.

[66] Clarkson, T. W. (1998). Human toxicology of mercury. J. Trace. Elem. Exp. Med., 11(2-3): 303-317.

[67] Dickman, M. D., and Leung, K. M. (1998). Mercury and Organochlorine exposure from fish consumption in Hong Kong. Chemosphere, 37(5): 991-1015.

[68] Olaifa, F. G, Olaifa, A. K, Onwude, T. E. (2004). Lethal and sublethal effects of copper to the African Cat fish (Clarias gariepnus). Afr. J. Biomed. Res., 7: 65-70.

[69] Bukola, D, Zaid, A, Olalekan, E. I, and Falilu, A. (2015). Consequences of anthropogenic activities on fish and the aquatic environment. *Poultry, Fisheries and Wildlife Sciences* 3: Article 138 (12 pp).

[70] Gillilan, D. C, and Brown, T. C. (1997). Instream flow protection. Washington, DC: Island Press.

[71] Rosenberg, D. M, Mccully, P, and Pringle, C. M. (2000). Global-scale environmental effect of hydrological alteration: Introduction. BioScience 50: 746-751.

[72] Wilcove, D. S, Rothstein, D, Dubow, J, Philips, A, and Losos, E. (1998). Quantifying threats to imperiled species in the United States. BioScience 48: 607-615.

[73] Abolude, D. S., Davies, O. A., and Avong, D.W. (2009). Level of heavy metals in freshwater crab (Cardisoma guahumi) obtained from Ahmadu Bello University Reservoir, Zaria, Nigeria. International Journal of Animal and Veterinary Advances 1: 54-58.

[74] Ayodele, J. T, and Abubakar, M. (2001). Chromium and copper in water, sediments and their bioaccumulation by freshwater bivalves in Tiga Lake, Nigeria. Journal of Environmental Sciences 5: 177-184.

[75] Kang, X, Mu, S, Li, W, and Zhao, N. (2012). Toxic effects of cadmium on crabs and shrimps. In: Acree W (ed.), Toxicity and drug testing. InTech (www.intechopen.com). pp 221-236.

[76] Sheriff, M. K, Awadallah, R. M, and Mohamed, A. E. (1979). Determination of trace elements of Egyptian crops by INAA. Journal of Radioanalytical Chemistry 53: 145-151.

[77] Swarnalatha, K, Letha, J, and Ayoob, S. (2013), Ecological risk assessment of a tropical lake system. Journal of Urban and Environmental Engineering 7: 323-329.

[78] Tay, C. K, Asmah, R, and Biney, C. A. (2009). Trace metal levels in water and sediment from the Sakumo II and Muni Lagoons, Ghana. West African Journal of Applied Ecology 16: 75-94

[79] Bukar, H. and Sa'id, M. D. (2014). Determination of Some Heavy Metals in Selected Poultry Feeds Available in Kano Metropolis, Nigeria. *Chemistry Search Journal* Vol. 5(1), Pp 8-11.

[80] Koivo, L. and Oravainen, O. (1982). Inc in water and sediment of two lakes. Hydrobiologia 91:155-160.

[81] Szefer, P. and Szefer, S. Z. B. (1990). Distribution of trace metals in some representative fauna of the southern Baltic. Mar. Pollut. and Buttl. 26, 60-62.

[82] FAO. (2006). Livestock's long shadow: environmental issues and options, by H. Steinfeld, P. Gerber, T.

Wassenaar, V. Castel, M. Rosales and C. de Haan. Rome. (Available at http://www.virtualcentre.org/en/library/key_pub/longshad/a0701e/A0701E00.pdf).

[83] Burton, C. and Turner, C. (2003). Manure management: treatment strategies for sustainable agriculture, 2nd edition, Bedford, UK, Silsoe Research Institute.

[84] Farkas, A, Salanki, J, and Specziar, A. (2002). Relation between growth and the heavy metal concentration in organs of bream Abramis brama L. populating Lake Balaton. *Arch. Environ. Contam. Toxicol.*, 43(2): 236-243.

[85] Akanni, K. A., and Benson, O. B. (2014). Poultry Wastes Management Strategies and Environmental Implications on Human Health in Ogun State of Nigeria. Advances in Economics and Business, 2(4), 164-171.

[86] FAO (2008). Poultry waste management in developing countries Charles Michael Williams, North Carolina State University, Department of Poultry Science, Raleigh NC, United States of America

[87] Saad, M. M (2016). The risk of human exposure to antibiotic Residues from food of both animal and plant origin. EJBPS 3(5): 12-15.

[88] Chinivasagam, H. N, Redding, M, Runge, G, and Blackall, P. J. (2010). Presence And incidence of food borne pathogens in Australian chicken litter. Broiler and Poultry Science 51(3): 311-318.

[89] Wilkinson, K, Tee, E, Tomkins, R, Hepworth, G, and Premier, R (2011). Effect of heating and aging of poultry litter on the persistence of Enteric bacteria. Poultry Science 90(1): 10-18.

[90] Rich, G. and Cherry, K. (1987). Hazardous Waste Treatment Technologies Pudvan Publishers, New York